Total
Vision

TOTAL VISION

Richard S. Kavner, O.D.
Lorraine Dusky

Illustrations by Felice Gittelman

A & W VISUAL LIBRARY
NEW YORK

Grateful acknowledgments are made to the following for permission to quote
from copyrighted works:

Beadle, Muriel. *A Child's Mind*. Copyright © 1970 by Muriel Beadle. Reprinted by
permission of Doubleday & Company, Inc.
Green, Elmer and Alyce. *Beyond Biofeedback*. Copyright © 1977 by Elmer and
Alyce Green. Reprinted by permission of Delacorte Press/Seymour Lawrence.
The I Ching or Book of Changes. The Richard Wilhelm translation rendered into
English by Cary F. Baynes. Bollingen Series XIX. Copyright 1950, © 1967 by
Princeton University Press. Copyright renewed 1977. Reprinted by permission of
Princeton University Press.
Jung, Carl. *Modern Man in Search of a Soul*. Reprinted by permission of Harcourt
Brace Jovanovich, Inc.
Kepes, G. *Language of Vision*. Reprinted by permission of S. I. Hayakawa and
Paul Theobald & Co.
Ott, John. *Health & Light*. Copyright © 1973 John Ott. Reprinted by permission
of the Devin-Adair Company.
Samuels, Mike and Nancy. *Seeing With The Mind's Eye*. Copyright © 1975 Mike
Samuels and Nancy Samuels. Copublished by Random House and the Bookworks.
Reprinted by permission of the authors.
Some of the material in this book originally appeared in *Town & Country*
magazine.
Published by
A & W Publishers, Inc.
95 Madison Avenue
New York, New York 10016

Library of Congress Catalog Card Number: 79-6562
ISBN: 0-89104-181-8

Printed in the United States of America

To A. M. Skeffington

When many were satisfied with simple answers, he had the foresight to ask difficult questions and follow them up with diligent research.

Acknowledgments

There are many people who have helped me professionally through the years. I would like to thank some of them here.

Dr. Harold A. Solan, for teaching me what it means to be a professional.

Dr. William Ludlam, for teaching me that all patients deserve a chance no matter how difficult the prognosis.

Dr. Norman Haffner, for teaching me that all people deserve care whether or not they can afford it.

I would like to thank Felice Gittelman for the care and thought she put into the illustrations.

I would also like to thank my father and mother, Saul and Sylvia, and my wife and sons, Carole, Ted and Bill, for love and devotion through all the difficult hours.

—Richard Kavner

I used to think books were solo flights, but now I know the fallacy of that, and so I wish to thank several people for their help in getting this one airborne: John M. Baldwin, III for his encouragement from the beginning, his comments throughout and his editing at the end; John Duffy, for his 24-hour telephone service when I needed a piece of obscure information, both factual and metaphysical; Edward Tedeschi, for his time and thought; Barbara King, for putting up with me when our home became an office for several months; Diana Davenport, for her faith and support when I was down and out; Richard Kavner, my coauthor, for his patience, understanding and support, but most of all for his demonstration of the *camera obscura* on the night of the Blizzard of '78; and my editor, Angela Miller, who started the whole project when she said: "I went to a party, and when I took off my glasses I acted quite differently. . . ."

For their help on various and sundry parts of the book, I would like to thank Jerry Anderson, Cole Patterson, Edna Kucher, Neil Michelson and Rene Gladstone.

I would also like to say hello and thanks to my ninth-grade English teacher, Mrs. Brady, wherever she is; George Borovsky, whose encouragement goes back to at least when I was ten; and my mother, who for many years did not understand what I was doing with my life but who came to accept it and me with humor and love.

—Lorraine Dusky

Contents

Foreword

It is our belief that as patients we are too passive about our health and well-being. With scant—and sometimes incorrect—information we are often not able to make intelligent choices about the protection and enhancement of our vision. The pattern in the past has been to leave its development to chance, but because of the demands our technological culture places on vision, we maintain "development by chance" will no longer suffice. We cannot alter the situation; we can learn to have vision to meet the needs of the times. We can improve on our Stone Age eyes.

With this in mind, we are providing information from a wide variety of fields: optometry, nutrition, child development, psychology, neurology and physiology. All of these are related to our visual sense. Our hope is that an informed reader will make intelligent choices based on the advances in these areas to protect not only his or her own vision, but that of the generations to come.

However, each person is an individual with different needs at different times, and what may be helpful to one person may be detrimental to another. You should have a practitioner sensitive to your special needs and willing to discuss them with you. Good health or sickness is not an isolated event but relates to the whole individual.

We are also providing exercises for your eyes, not as a means of treating any specific problems, but as an introduction to how vision may be protected and enhanced and to teach you how to see in different ways.

We hope *Total Vision* will be a stepping stone to a lifetime of healthy vision.

Richard Kavner, O.D., and Lorraine Dusky

Introduction

Vision is much more than opening our eyes, the way one might turn on the television. The ability to comprehend what we see is a process involving the brain as well as the eyes, and it has developed through trial and error. The way Homo sapiens sees today is a result of his development through the ages; the way each individual sees is the product of his own development throughout his lifetime.

Vision is an active process which begins at birth and constantly undergoes minor shifts and alterations due to 1) a basic predisposition to a specific personality, evident at birth; 2) biochemical influences, or nutrition, and 3) the physical environment, including the actions of the parents.

The biochemical and physical climate does the first fine-tuning of our eyes and gives each one of us our own vision of the world. Even the food a child eats is a factor in determining the growth and development of his general abilities, specifically including his visual skills. When adequate vitamins and proteins are lacking, the art of seeing may be seriously impaired.

Also crucial to a child's development is the external physical environment—which includes everything from the attitudes of his parents to the location of their home. Unwittingly or knowingly, a parent may encourage some skills and downplay others; neither action is lost on the child, who usually will learn to adjust his actions in favor of the more acceptable behavior with which he and his family feel comfortable. However, a child may choose to revolt against these pressures, which sets up other difficulties. If the child is fortunate a parent may help him choose a more appropriate and less troublesome behavior. A healthy child will do whatever he has to in order to get the stimulation he needs to grow. If screaming works, so be it.

Many researchers have discovered that all children go through the same stages of development, which can be observed, codified and predicted. For example, the "terrible twos" is a phase most children and their sometimes exasperated parents will probably experience. Not so easily observable are the changing perceptual stages of a child's life, when he first experiences his environment and then settles back to comprehend it.

As he grows, a period of expansiveness and receptivity to the world around him is followed by a time of intense internalizing as the child makes sense of what he has experienced. That completed to his satisfaction, he moves to another phase of openness. This occurs throughout life.

Development is determined by how the child, in his own genetically determined style, responds to each phase, and how others—mother, father, sisters, brothers and even Aunt Jennie—respond to him. If the child meets some resistance to his behavior along the way, and the obstacle is repeated again and again, he will at first experience a sense of disequilibrium, or stress. In his own way he will decide either to *fight* the obstacle and grope for other responses or take *flight* from it, discontinuing the action which brings disapproval or discomfort. In accommodating the obstacle he may distort his behavior, such as tilt his head away from it, or simply not perceive it at all. In such a manner a child may continually block vision in one eye so that eventually, through months or years of repetition, he becomes "blind" in one eye; his method of dealing with a certain stress is to ignore it.

All human responses, vision included, exist because of their survival value to the individual and the species. Man's eyes originally developed to look out into the distance and search the horizon for animals —not to spend hours each day focusing at near point, which is the way of the world today in literate cultures. More than likely, as we become students of the printed word, we adapt the eyes to meet the stress. Unless we periodically and frequently relax, look out the window and focus at a distance, we may end up distorting our optical system. The stress on our ancient optics is the reason that the more educated you are, the more likely it is that you wear glasses. In effect, nearsighted eyes have learned not to bother with distance.

The eyes are so interrelated with the mind that a visual examination can often be a means of looking backward to learn which life choices a person has made—consciously or unconsciously—and what stresses he has encountered along the way. In an examination by a vision therapist you will certainly be asked to read letters on a chart, but that's only the beginning.

Vision therapy includes a series of exercises which will help an individual unlearn many inappropriate responses. It is a means of helping a person develop healthy vision, undistorted and flexible enough to meet all of today's needs—to read a book or spot a horse on the horizon.

Vision therapy is not done to the patient; the therapist merely arranges the conditions which allow a person to learn the appropriate responses and integrate them into an acceptable and comfortable way of being. Vision therapy is not a system designed to do away with eyeglasses, although for some that may be the result. Vision therapy is an experience in perception. Its aim: seeing everything.

———

The quotes at the beginning of each chapter are from the *I Ching*.

For the sake of clarity, the male gender is used throughout the book to denote both sexes rather than the his/her construction.

1
What Is Vision Therapy?

However men may differ in disposition and in education,
the foundations of human nature are the same in everyone.

"Do you understand?" he asked.

"Yes, I see," she replied.

Such overlapping of meaning in language is not simply an acci-
dent—it undoubtedly is the result of early man's perception that vision
and comprehension are delicately interwoven. But as science attempted
to explain eyesight with diagrams resembling some sort of Kodak in our
eyeballs, the concept that sight is related to insight got lost in the new
technology that permeated our thinking in the last century. The time
has come to revise this attitude, for now we can explain and put into
practice an idea which has been around since at least Socrates: Vision
is not only what we see, but also what we are prepared to perceive.

And since perception is the *aha!* that occurs in our head whenever
memory and intuition are integrated with new data, it makes sense
that impaired vision scrambles the data and skews the perception. The
alarming news is that a great number of us—perhaps as many as 70
percent—have visual inefficiencies of which we are not even aware.

In the last half century a new science called behavioral optometry
—the combined knowledge of psychology, neurology, biology, child
development and other related fields—has given us a concept of vision
that is probably what our ancestors intuitively sensed but could not
explain: Our eyes are receptors of the brain. The eyes take in the data,
channels them along neural impulses to the cortex, where the central control makes sense out of them and we see images: meadows and mountains, Aunt Jean and the boy who delivers your newspaper, the sheep-
dog who lives next door, the numbers in your checkbook and a green

1

magnum of champagne. As you read those words, your mind probably conjured up images which came into view and departed in the twinkling of an eye.

Vision, therefore, is no mere passive occurrence such as breathing, but is instead a complex and learned process which occurs mainly in the brain. The way we think affects our vision, and our vision affects the way we think: *What we see is how we are, and how we are determines what we see.* And if that's the case, then by improving our visual skills, much as we can improve coordination of other parts of the body, we can realize an expanded perspective or vision, as it were, of the world. Conversely, impaired visual skills narrow our field of vision and limit our perspective, sometimes leaving in their wake bizarre symptoms which seemingly have nothing to do with sight. But through vision therapy, which teaches the eye/brain system to operate smoothly, efficiently and up to its potential, the resulting changes permit the individual to "see" and act differently.

Sometimes remarkable psychological changes accompany better vision, as the following examples illustrate:

A 9-year-old youngster who was thought to be retarded had been in special classes for three years. He seemed doomed never to progress beyond the simplest educational and vocational abilities. A New York City school guidance counselor who knew of this new approach to vision recommended that the boy be given a complete examination. What showed up was a fusion problem. Although the youngster was seeing with each eye, he was unable to coordinate both eyes smoothly. This caused the information taken in to be jumbled, giving him severe perceptual problems in organizing his thoughts. He began a program of therapy with weekly visits and training to be done at home and at school. After two difficult and frustrating years he tested at normal intelligence and transferred to regular school classes. That was 10 years ago. Today he is an accounting student in college.

A teenager with severe strabismus—crossed eyes—was failing in high school and eventually dropped out. He drifted around the country for a few years and eventually returned home to Long Island. Unable to find a job he could handle, he stayed home and was for all practical purposes a cripple. His demeanor vacillated from agitated to dejected. He had no social life.

At 20 he began psychoanalysis, and his therapist suggested vision therapy for his crossed eye, believing that by "looking in" so intensely he was blocking out much of the world. The young man insisted that the problem was "all in my head." As a child, he had tried a program of exercises to strengthen the eye muscles and correct the crossed eye, but to little or no avail. Eventually, however, he agreed to have his eyes tested.

As a patient, he was irritable and immature in his demands—he wanted appointments set up and changed at whim. If things didn't go his way, he acted as if he were being persecuted.

During a summer of training, his eyes began to straighten. He kept it up for a year until his strabismus totally disappeared, but by then he was making life hell for his psychotherapist. Without a physical problem which demanded others give him special treatment, he became self-indulgent and capricious. Eventually this attitude broke down, and his outlook improved markedly. He decided to finish high school. When he entered college, he qualified for a scholarship, and received his very first A. Semi-annual examinations show that he has retained his hard-won improvements.

A 16-year-old student in a family of achievers worked hard at her schoolwork but continually received low grades. Her physical coordination made her a last choice for team games. Then she started blacking out during tests. A standard eye examination rated her acuity 20/20, but when referred to a Washington, D.C., specialist, it was discovered that she had poor eye coordination, usually the result of stress created by the use of the eyes for intense close work.

After a year of therapy her grades improved from Ds to Bs. In her freshman year at college the teenager who had always worried about scholastic probation made the honors list. Her physical coordination improved markedly.

Enthusiastic about her therapy, she worked as an aide in the doctor's office, helping to keep eight or 10 patients at a time working on different tasks. She now talks about vision therapy at every opportunity. Her name: Luci Johnson Nugent.

"The key to a better education is better vision," says the former President's daughter. "If you don't have that key, you can't open the door to a better life."

These case studies may sound amazing when you consider that they are the outcome of a type of training which at first glance appears to be no more than eye exercises. But they are easily understandable once you stop thinking of the eye as a camera and consider it a part—albeit an important one—of the entire visual apparatus which begins and ends at the back of the brain, where we interpret electrochemical messages from our ever-changing world.

Good vision is much more than acuity, which only refers to how clearly you can see. It involves a whole spectrum of skills: How well can you use both eyes together? How quickly can you judge left from right? How well do you see objects in space? Can you shift focus from near to far quickly and easily? How good is your visual memory? How easily can you change your point of view? Are your visual skills equal to your age? Your needs?

A behavioral examination checks all the above and more. Yet at the present time most routine examinations just check for disease and test acuity on a chart that is over a hundred years old. You may do remarkably well reading those little letters and be disease free, but you can still be walking around with a load of hidden visual problems which can do anything from making you cranky or rigid in your outlook, giving you a backache or making you seem less intelligent than you are. You may know you've got good ideas in your head, but you just can't seem to get them out. And the blocked passageway could be an inefficient visual system.

The basic premise of vision therapy is that vision is learned. Since that is so, we can learn how to see properly—if we've been doing anything wrong—with guidance. Vision therapy is not a program to strengthen, enlarge, shrink or change eye muscles—which, by the way, are a lot stronger than they need be to do their job—but simply a method to teach the entire visual system *including the brain* to operate at peak efficiency.

In the process a person's psychological makeup, which may be both cause and effect of visual problems, often undergoes basic changes. But it's not a one-way street: Visual problems may cause psychological and emotional difficulties, and psychological disturbances could cause visual problems. In any event, they may reflect each other, but this does not mean that psychological problems are always linked to vision.

A youngster in grade school quickly learns that intense concentration on his books brings the kind of achievement valued in our culture: good grades. But eyes not equipped to handle the job can keep him from being able to learn through reading. If he falls behind his peers, he develops certain feelings about himself and emotional problems stemming from the frustration of failure. By the time he's a teenager, the emotional difficulty has a life of its own and is likely to be imbedded in personality and behavior.

Vision therapy can teach his eyes to operate more efficiently and thereby seemingly unlock several IQ points, but the behavior stemming from all those years when he felt stupid is probably not going to clear up overnight, or perhaps ever. He's practiced his responses, no matter whether they're pleasant or not. Behavior is well rehearsed and committed to memory, to feelings, to muscle.

But enhancing or expanding vision can and often does change personality and behavior, because in the process an individual acquires better tools to understand himself and to perceive the world around him and where he fits into the grand scheme of life. To the uninitiated the idea may sound farfetched, but it fits neatly into the current understanding of how the body and brain operate as a single unit, with each sphere having effect on the other.

Biologists and psychologists from several schools—Reichian on through the various types of massage, movement and megavitamin therapies—believe that our physical being does not operate in a vacuum separate from our mental being. For instance, it was recently learned that spring fever is not just a case of lassitude brought on by the fact that when the skies are blue the living should be easy. The general tiredness one feels is the result of the body working to absorb all that additional Vitamin D you are getting as you sit in the sun. Several studies indicate that the emotional whirlwind many women experience in the days preceding their menstrual period can be brought under control to some extent by increasing their intake of the B vitamins, especially B_6.

What all this means is that each thought or state of mind has a biological component, and each physical action or internal biological condition has a psychological effect. Thus every muscle movement has a psychological response, and vice versa. For example, a cat brushing up against your legs can either feel silky and pleasant or cause you to shudder slightly and step back. Of course, many physical responses have scant effect upon our psychological makeup, at least in the normal order of things, but with a sensation as encompassing and important as seeing—that sense which has more brain connections than any other —the input-output is critical.

Then there is the work of Dr. Hans Selye, the renowned stress expert at the University of Montreal, who showed that all living things— and thus all parts of the body—either adapt to prolonged stress or die. An organ, such as your heart, that is violently exercised will either strengthen or completely break down; a person who lives in extreme cold undergoes increased thyroid activity to produce more internal heat and develops a layer of body fat. All this is directed by the central intelligence center of the brain, which receives information, analyzes it and sends back commands. A drop in skin temperature informs the brain that it is cold outside, and the brain automatically decides to step up thyroid activity to turn up your thermostat.

The eyes are no exception. In effect, focusing at near point for prolonged periods of time, as we do when we read, is actually a signal to the brain to fix the focus in that position—that is, become nearsighted. The eyes have accommodated the stress of reading hour after hour by changing to be more comfortable seeing up close than at a distance. It could be said that the scholar who wants to spend his life among books is really adapting to his career if he becomes nearsighted. Of course, something had to give, and that is usually his distance vision. Not surprisingly, people in cultures who primarily use their distance vision are generally farsighted.

Vision therapy, instead of dealing with the symptoms the way glasses do, gets at the root of the problem, and that is why the changes in behavior can be so profound. Although some people who undergo training may end up no longer needing glasses, and indeed this may be the reason you picked up this book, our aim is much more than that. Vision therapy offers a means of protecting and enhancing your vision, and particularly that of the next generation.

Man evolved in the mountains and plains, and his eyes developed to look out into the distance so that he could hunt. We no longer need that skill, but it is certainly worth our while to preserve our distance vision and help our eyes adapt to city life and its different visual panorama.

A full 50 percent of the population today wears glasses for something more than keeping out the sun. Contrast that with the fact that only between two and three percent of us are born with visual deformities. But because we have become convinced that the commonest eye defects are hereditary and thus largely unchangeable, we accept the idea that there is basically nothing we can do to change the situation. To the contrary, considerable research indicates it is unlikely that the breakdown is programmed into the species; it is solid evidence that we are doing something to cause it.

The Eye Is Not a Camera
While advances in other branches of medicine have moved forward dramatically in recent years, eye care has stagnated except for the re-

finement of surgical procedures. The average nearsighted child, for instance, is handed spectacles similar to those worn in Ben Franklin's day and is told he can look forward to a life behind glasses. The reason is that we have unfortunately been misled into thinking of the eye as a camera, a misconception which restricted research and modes of treatment.

The idea was that light comes through the pupil, is bent by the lens, and comes to a point of focus on the retina, where the image is. According to this theory, the smaller the image, the clearer the picture.

But this concept is far removed from what actually happens in the visual system. If you were given a camera with all the built-in distortions and imperfections of the eye, you would be back at the store demanding that your money be returned as soon as you had shot your first roll of film.

Let us consider the "perfect" eye:

—There is no single point of focus for any image, even when we wear proper glasses that give us 20/20 vision. The eye is constructed so that rays of light which enter through the center of the lens are not bent, but the ones above, below, right and left are. The farther you go from the center of the lens, the greater the bending. Thus, light rays which come from an object will be bent at varying degrees, depending upon where they enter the eye. Those at the center will be bent the least, those at the periphery will be bent the most. The image is then spread over an *area* and not focused on a single point.

Although it is true that when a pupil contracts the scattering will be reduced, it will not be totally eliminated. Interestingly enough, the smallest part of the bundle of light rays does not give the clearest picture. An area other than the smallest is clearer. This can be demonstrated to yourself with a magnifying glass. As you adjust the glass, for instance, you will find that the smallest image does not give the clearest picture. The image will appear fuzzy, clear up as you move the glass closer, and then fuzz up again.

—An eye has uncorrected color distortion. That different colors have different wavelengths was demonstrated by Sir Isaac Newton more than three centuries ago when he showed that light passing through a prism is broken up into the colors of the rainbow. These light waves travel at different speeds and come to focus differently. Blue comes to focus first and red last. In a camera, this would give a blurred image, with colors slopping from one object to another.

Yet we see an integrated image of colors, unaware that the color bands are activated in different times and places. What has happened

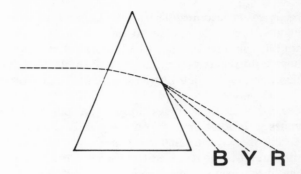

The chromatic parts of the visual spectrum are evident when light passes through a prism and the colors of the spectrum become visible.

is that farther along the way—somewhere in the computer of the brain —these impulses are put together so that we see a single image with the colors neatly filled in.

Experiments show that when you eliminate this distortion, or *chromatic aberration,* people lose their ability to focus their eyes accurately. It appears that it is a necessary part of the proper functioning of the perfect eye. Perhaps it operates as a feedback system to help the eye adjust for clarity in a manner similar to a self-focusing camera, for when we focus on an object, this mechanism oscillates in and out until

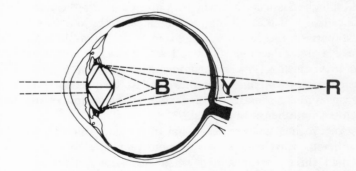

The eye's chromatic spectrum: The lens of the eye acts as a double prism from base to base. Light which enters the eye emerges from the lens divided into a spectrum of colors from blue to red. Each color travels at a different speed and comes to a focus at a different point. In the normal eye, the yellow-green focus is usually on the retina.

it settles on a particular focus, the way we adjust a radio dial for the clearest sound.

—A perfect eye continually wiggles. You know what happens when you don't hold the camera still: fuzzy pictures. Well, the eye is in constant motion, oscillating from side to side. This slight but constant movement is normally imperceptible. In one experiment, a special contact lens was rigged up to keep the image stabilized as if the eye did not move. Within a minute, the subject experienced a loss of vision. Some believe that the oscillating, or *physiological nystagmus,* is a method of preventing our eyes from becoming fixed to a single image and fatigued. On the other hand, it may be a process like chromatic aberration, a necessary feedback process to allow for fine visual tuning.

What we can glean from this is that the eye needs to be always on the go, looking here, looking there, picking out what it wants, what it can't help noticing, and shuffling all this information around. Perhaps it is a part of the way our "stream of consciousness" changes without our doing anything conscious about it: New information keeps coming in and moving around the old.

This constant ebb and flow is undoubtedly part of the way we adapt to the ever-changing schema of life. Become "fixed" on something to the exclusion of new data, and you lose your perspective. Intellectually we may have lost the comprehension connection to sight, but language kept it intact through the years.

If the eye is not a camera, can the retina operate as film? Obviously not.

To begin with, the retina is constructed in such a way that it appears to be backwards. Its sensitive elements, the rods and cones, face away from the light coming in through the pupil. Not only that, but light which travels through the inside of the eye to the rear of the retina must pass through layers of nerve cells, fibers and vessels before it finally stimulates the rods and cones.

Light is absorbed by the visual pigment, rhodopsin, which then stimulates the rods and cones to send an electrochemical charge— *backwards* to the front of the eye. Many such impulses gather there and are combined at the optic nerve, which sends its messages toward the back of the eye again and on to the visual centers of the brain. A seemingly roundabout way of doing business.

Most of us consider the retina to be like film because it appears logical that each place which is stimulated forms an impression either at the retina or is relayed back to a specific area in the brain. However,

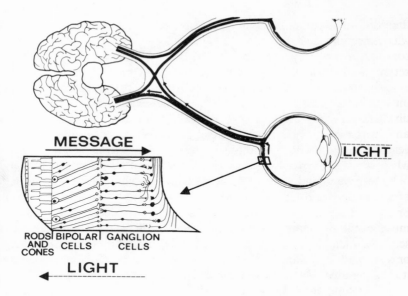

The visual message: Light enters the eye and is converted into an electric-chemical code in the retina. This code is carried along the optic nerve to the higher visual centers for interpretation, verification and classification.

if we look closely at the retina, we find that the construction of the tissue would not allow this simplistic concept. Almost every rod and cone has its message gathered by another cell, called a bipolar cell. Each bipolar cell acts as a central receiving station for a group of rods and cones.

At times a cone will share its information with a bipolar cell as well as send it directly to the higher visual centers in the cortex. In effect, the bipolar cells act like funnels, for there are many more rods and cones than bipolar cells. These way stations start a process of sorting out information so that it can be sent on in fewer categories. There are also horizontal cells which do no more than connect bipolar cells to other bipolar cells, sometimes over rather long distances, rather than to those right next door.

As a matter of fact, one bipolar cell may actually influence the visual message of another. It's a process of refinement. The stimulation of the rods and cones will therefore not necessarily be the same message as it leaves the bipolar cells. This same refinement of information is seen at the next level of the retina, where several bipolar cells send their information on to ganglion cells. In turn, these are connected with other ganglion cells. To add to this refinement process, we have some fibers which come directly from the brain's visual centers to the retina—a one-way hot line to control the action.

It is possible that in this inner mix, the original rod and cone impulse has been lost, modified or changed to suit the needs of the individual, for that appears to be the function of the retina. The analysis and refinement of light on the retina is under the control of the higher centers of the brain, and this makes our visual apparatus—a part of which is the eyeball—much more like a computer than a camera.

The eye is used as a converter of light energy to carry out a process of analyzing what has already been initiated by the visual centers in the brain, so that we only see what we are willing and ready to see. Nothing more, nothing less. The brain makes a decision about what there is to see, and then uses the visual system and other senses either to deny or confirm this hypothesis. The conclusion is called perception, and it is no wonder that each person's is different.

So what appear to be deficiencies if the eye were a camera are actually the intricate mechanisms for transmitting information to the mind. The brain acts like a wise old sage who listens to all his messengers, the senses, before he conjures up an image, a thought, a perception. Of course, this sage receives information at a speed approaching 300 miles per hour, and so makes to us what seems like a lot of snap decisions.

The eye has three other functions besides providing form perception, which is what we have been talking about. Approximately 20 percent of the information from the retina never goes to the visual cortex to be used for sight, but instead travels to other brain centers to be integrated with more data about the body's orientation and position in space. This function guides us as we move about, and it appears to be a much older system than form perception, for we must be oriented to our environment before we can identify other creatures and objects.

The retina also uses light to stimulate the pineal and pituitary glands, the master glands of the body which regulate the entire system. Although we are just beginning to learn about this process, it is thought that light causes the glands to produce certain hormones necessary for our well-being. The rays of the sun appear to be a necessary nutrient, a fact many of us instinctively know as we dream of sunny beaches in February.

This light stimulation also seems to be related to fertility and may be the reason the seasons are related to the mating of animals. In spring, when the days of light are long, a young buck's thoughts turn to sex.*

Furthermore, the eyes appear to be critical to the development of affection. Eye contact with the primary care-giver, usually Mom, informs a child that he is related to another human being, which lets him know he is a member of a social group. This bonding may be critical for the survival of the species. Although the other senses, of course, complement this, when eye contact is denied or impossible, it seems to seriously hamper relationships with others throughout a person's life. Children who are blind from birth have an exceedingly difficult time giving and receiving affection.

Since we have been stuck with the concept of the eye as a camera for so long, it was also easy to believe that just the way we can change the image visible in a view finder by changing the lens, we could also fix up our sight by popping on a pair of lenses and letting it go at that. The traditional approach to eyes in trouble is glasses which change the bend of light rays coming in to accommodate the problem.

In effect, such glasses are like a crutch for a turned ankle; certainly they help you get around, but eventually you want to get rid of them and get your own appendage in fine working order. And consider how quickly a leg muscle atrophies when it has not been in circulation for a few weeks; eyes take longer to weaken, but the same principle applies. Naturally, for some, glasses will continue to be a necessary and useful aid to seeing clearly. Unfortunately, traditional medicine and the old way of thinking about our eyes as a fixed—and not fluid—sense got us into the habit of thinking of prescription lenses as the only treatment possible.

Yet vision therapy makes use of some types of lenses, or it may help an individual to understand better how and when to use his glasses. In some cases, and if the problem is caught early enough, it may prevent the need for glasses altogether. However, people who are near-

* Some animals, such as iguanas, retain a vestigal "third eye" on the top of their heads, which is thought to have been used to note the degree of heat of the sun, ergo, the season. In man, it is believed that this remnant of our evolutionary past dropped inside our skull and became the pineal gland. A tumor here can cause highly erratic sexual development.

sighted and want to eliminate the need to use their glasses constantly have more difficulty. Often lenses of a different sort are prescribed for people with special needs, such as those who do a lot of near-point work. Preventive lenses will help an individual relax his focus while seeing at near point and will counterbalance the stress such sight involves. These lenses are only needed for close work, and are less cumbersome than regular "nearsighted" glasses, which leave the bridges of some noses only when the lights go out.

Sometimes training lenses will be used in vision therapy to exaggerate a procedure and may no longer be needed after treatment.

Leaving aside the question of whether one will wear glasses or not, the results of vision therapy are encouraging: 75 percent of the people with crossed eyes and 85 percent of the children with vision-related learning disabilities are treated successfully. While almost everybody sees better to some degree after therapy, a full 50 percent will show a difference that is measurable—letters on the eye chart you couldn't read before you will now rattle off with ease. Distant signs will be easier to read. And 15 percent will actually show a change in the eye's measurements, a modification which previously was not thought possible.

This is particularly important today, for the statistics show that we are becoming a generation of the visually handicapped: Nearsightedness, astigmatism and the hidden visual problems, such as coordination and perceptual difficulties related to eye inefficiencies, are all on the rise.

Nearsightedness goes hand in hand with literacy, for the amount of time spent focusing at near point is directly related to myopia. What could this mean to the gestalt of the times? If we are nearsighted, we tend to concentrate on only that which is near—and no one's closer to ourselves than our own psyche. That could be the reason that we have been coined the "me generation," with our emphasis on personality, introspection and the question, *How will this affect me?* prefacing everything we do.

It could turn out that this generation's perspective is too narrow, too limiting, too nearsighted. It is at least interesting to note that some philosophers have an eye which turns out and appear to be gazing off into the distance rather than focusing on the here and now.

Vision Therapy Began with the Greeks

Vision therapy and what it promises is based on the premise of psychobiology, a relatively new science which proposes that what happens *in the mind* occurs simultaneously—but differently—*in the body*. The idea of a "sound mind in a sound body" goes back to the ancient Greeks, but only in the last half century have the pieces of the puzzle showing how this works begun to fit together.

The foundations and history of vision therapy are intertwined with developments in a number of fields—science and medicine, philosophy and art, religion and education. In all of these we know that each person's perception is different. If three people witness an event and relate what happened later, there will be three different versions.

Physical causes for mental disturbances have been sought since earliest times, and as late as 1881 the *Encyclopaedia Britannica* classified insanity as a disease of the brain inducing mental symptoms. Even Freud, whose theories of psychoanalysis were responsible for making many of those who came after him denigrate the mind/body connection, himself characterized schizophrenia as biochemical in origin and predicted that one day we would have a chemical cure for it.

But what happened in modern times was that the advance of science brought with it the attitude that all phenomena must be capable of being verified by observation or experiment, or they did not exist; and since science or philosophy could not empirically prove the connection between mind and body, we tended to dismiss the premise. Many still do today.

But the concept that perception is the result of a dynamic interaction between the individual and the world was kept alive in philosophy and education. In medicine, the belief that visual problems were either mechanical failures or accidents of birth came to be commonly accepted. In the last 30 years or so, research has delved into the mysteries of the visual process and in doing so has inadvertently discovered that this interaction between individual and world is actually how the visual system develops into its adult form. A baby's vision and perception, just like the rest of his body and brain, are vastly different from what they will be when he grows up.

What recent research has shown is that while we are born with a given set of nerves and muscles, these must be nourished in a compatible environment to meet the taxing demands of our culture. In effect, these advances at the forefront of science, medicine, philosophy and education have brought us full circle to what some early philosophers believed. Only now we're learning how things work.

The idea that sight can be improved can be traced to the early Egyptians who treated crossed eyes with a mask which had eye holes set far apart. An inward turning eye would be forced to look out to see, and although the treatment sounds crude, it could work.

A thousand or so years later the Greeks came along and set down the basic principles of scientific thought. They said first what we still debate today: Perception occurs when man interacts in some way with his environment. What is perceived depends not only upon the nature of the object, but on the nature of the observer as well. And since man is constantly changing, his perception does also.

Believing in a changing and imperfect world, the Greeks knew our own perceptions of it could only be approximations of reality. Just as a referee at the Super Bowl will tell you, what I see is different from what you see, and what is real is something else again.

The surgeon in attendance to Socrates and friends was Alcmaeon, who was, to put it mildly, ahead of his times. From his animal and human dissections he concluded that the eye was connected to the brain by certain pathways (today we call them nerves) and theorized that visual sensations came together there, where they integrated with memory and thought. Misperception, he wrote, was due to a clogging of these channels. Although today we know a lot more about what happens where in the body, our centuries of searching are slowly bringing us back to what Alcmaeon knew: Physiology and psychology are not independent sciences.

Recent knowledge of brain development and function has shown intelligence to be fixed by heredity, to a certain degree, yet malleable by forces within the environment. By recognizing that life is a dynamic equilibrium, a give and take which occurs between the individual and his surroundings, contemporary scientists have shown that intelligence, and even the architecture of the brain, can be influenced.

Animal research has shown that the greater the interaction with the environment, the greater the quantity and quality of the brain tissue.

During the Dark Ages between the fall of Rome and the Renaissance, St. Augustine stood out as one of the few innovative voices. He proposed that a willing mind is necessary before learning can prosper, no matter how rich the environment. Augustine, a colorful fourth-century character, may have picked this up by reflecting on his own life, for although he was raised by a pious mother, he was rather a rake until he decided it was time to change his ways; practically overnight he became a champion of the Church. Now we use words such as motivation and desire, and understand that it is not enough to leave a child in a roomful of educational toys and shut the door; the toys will not educate. It is the interaction between child and toy that does.

An Arab named Al Hazen made the next important discovery in our story. About 1000 A.D. he demonstrated that light is bent, or refracted, when it travels through different substances. It took 300 years more for someone to put that knowledge to use and invent spectacles.

While Roger Bacon's invention will always be a boon to mankind, the spectacles did have the effect of endorsing the mind/body split by separating *insight* from sight. Put on a pair of them and *presto!* you can see better. What else could be involved? We began thinking of the eye as a dandy little unit, basically independent of thinking and comprehension, which could be patched up, when in trouble, with glasses, and later, drugs and surgery. Correcting vision became solely a medical problem. The comprehensive connection—that relationship between sight and insight—was forgotten.

Another influence which separated sight from perception even more was the invention of a device called a *camera obscura* in the 1600s. Through a tiny hole in a darkened box, one could reflect a mirror image of an object or a person onto the opposite surface. The large image had amazingly passed through a tiny opening. Not only was the contraption a source of fascination in the drawing room, it made it all the easier to believe that the eye was somehow a similar device: If light could pass through a small opening and reconstruct an image, wasn't it likely the same thing happened in the eye?

At the same time, medical men were dissecting the brain and the nervous system and proclaiming that all that was necessary for everyone to see the same way was undamaged tissue and responsive muscles. The message of the philosophers who held that different men must see differently was lost.

Christianity was at least partially responsible for the attitude that philosophy, which dealt with the mind, and science, which dealt with the body, should be treated as two distinctly separate spheres. Inherent in Christian dogma is the concept of a disembodied soul which is usually depicted at war with man's baser element, the flesh.

Pre-Reformation scientists who served up theories seemingly at odds with this idea were excommunicated—no small concern in the days when religion was enmeshed in every aspect of life. Descartes stands alone as one who meticulously accounted for the separate domains of spirit and body and thereby escaped the Catholic Church's denunciation.

Now, since a scientist had once been a child, after all, and was likely to have had a religious upbringing, the impact of his early experiences on his intellectual inquiry cannot be discounted. We can never quite eradicate the influences of our youth, even if we make an effort to.

But others besides the Christians accepted the mind/body split. The idea was prevalent in all cultures and religions, including Judaism, which teaches that the way to wisdom is to question the nature of man.

To avoid the whole issue of the mind/body problem, scientific inquiry about man proceeded along two divergent lines: One group delved into the psyche and the subconscious, and the other into the physical and observable. Rarely did the twain meet. Indeed, the furor Darwin's theory of evolution caused was due to the fact that man, apart from all other living things, was theoretically imbued with something extra—a soul—and now here was this heretic saying we could all be traced to animal origins. Today we know how close we are to our primitive background. The cerebral cortex, thought to be the seat of our higher intellect, is a layer of cells no thicker than a matchbook. It wraps around our pre-human brain.

We lost sight of the fact that a whole group of people—the philosophers—kept telling us in different voices that man is a sort of continuum from the abstract to the real, that feelings and perceptions of this world do not exist apart from the minutiae of the millions of cells which go into the being of a single body.

What the seventeenth-century philosophers Spinoza and Locke had to say sounds not unlike the message of the Greeks: Spinoza postulated that what we see is not a copy of what exists, it is highly dependent upon our previous experiences, and thus perception is affected by memory, judgement and reason. Locke stated that only through the experiences of the senses do we acquire knowledge.

Spinoza also theorized that mind and body could not be separated into different spheres of being since they are one and the same. By the time he wrote that Spinoza had been excommunicated by the rabbis and forced to live on the outskirts of Amsterdam, where he supported himself as a polisher of lenses, dealing physically with the perception about which he theorized. Locke fared somewhat better, but had to leave England several times because of his opposition to the Catholicism of the reigning English monarchy. Their work, like their lives, sets them apart. Both men are examples of how their perceptions were the cause and effect of their experiences.

While science was teaching us more precisely how to turn fuzzy edges into sharp ones with lenses, an Irish cleric postulated in his *Essay*

Toward a New Theory of Vision that what is perceived is due to more than simply the optics of the individual. Bishop George Berkeley, the same mind that brought us the question of whether a tree falling in the forest makes a sound if there is no one within earshot, proposed that the only things which are real are our ideas about them, which spring from the information the senses process. What is seen is a subjective, personal impression, not necessarily an objective copy of the world.

In the same century ideas about personal freedom and human dignity would lead to revolutions in America and France, and these ultimately would advance the idea that man, the noble savage, could be improved, given a chance for education.

Considering that monarchs up to that point ruled by divine right, this thought reeked of treason, for, if you give a man the right to think for himself, he may no longer want someone to tell him what to decide.

The writings of an eighteenth-century philosopher and social theorist, Jean Jacques Rousseau, espoused the belief that expression rather than repression would produce free thinkers and educated men and women: Experience rather than analysis was the way to learn.

It was necessary to employ these principles to tame and civilize the "Wild Boy of Aveyron," a youth of approximately 11 who was thought to have been raised by wolves. Hunters had captured this strange and savage creature, human in appearance, animal in action. His care was entrusted to a physician at a school for the deaf, Jean Itard.

He surmised that the youth was uncivilized because he had not developed his senses along human lines. Itard decided first to try to reach the boy through touch, taste and smell; sight and hearing would come later. The doctor hoped that as the senses developed, so would intellect, and, in time, emotion, to add up to one complete person.

In five years Victor, as he came to be called, learned how to write and communicate his needs to others, but he was never able to speak. Itard had succeeded, at least to a degree, in reaching the mind through the senses.

Later the idea that learning occurs through the senses imprinting on the mind was expanded to encompass all mentally retarded children. A hundred years later Maria Montessori in Italy would start out working with the retarded and end up believing that the philosophy of learning by doing should be extended to all young children.

Here in the United States an educator, John Dewey, stated that children would learn best if they had a hand in deciding what and how to learn, and at what pace. In other words, when the children themselves decide to interact with their surroundings, they would learn best. It was the philosophy of St. Augustine dressed up in modern language and served to the school children of twentieth-century America.

In the field of psychology the thread of man's uniqueness was kept alive by Freud and Jung, who discussed the differences between each of us and how we got to be that way. An American, William James, felt that the nature of one's "stream of consciousness" resulted in a highly personal and ever-changing perception, and that perception is continually altered by the subjective awareness of the individual. James said that this kaleidoscopic stream of thoughts is the way we adapt to the surroundings. In other words, as the environment changes, so must we; it is the way we survive.

Back on the continent, the Gestalt school added that perception is a matter of organizing the incoming information and is the way an individual copes with his surroundings. How one perceives and copes are always in flux.

If the philosophers, and later the psychologists, have been saying all along that perception varies and is open to suggestion, why does this premise, which forms the foundation of vision therapy, sound so strange to our ears? For starters, there was the division between insight and sight, which is still prevalent; and furthermore, up to now there was no practical way of putting this knowledge to use. The biologists would show us the way.

A Russian physiologist, Ivan Pavlov, provided the basis for the concept that behavior is the result of the conditions of our life and largely a response to repetition of an act or event. What Pavlov did in his famous experiment was condition animals to respond to various stimuli, providing an explanation of how habits are formed: by repeating an act until it becomes a "conditioned reflex," integrated into behavior *without thinking about it.*

These concepts would ultimately lead to a new method of treatment for crossed eyes called *orthoptics,* based on the premise that a muscle's response can be reconditioned when strengthened by exercise.

But we propose that it is not the muscle alone which becomes conditioned, but the brain as well. It is the brain which acquires the bad habit, as it were, and directs the eye to do the wrong thing, such as turn in. For an eye to uncross and see straight, the reprogramming must occur in the brain.

Modern vision therapy bases its treatment for crossed eyes on this principle, and the current rate of success for this disturbing affliction is 75 percent. Yet surgery, which ideally results in two cosmetically straight eyes and the smooth, easy functioning of them as a working team, is successful only 20 percent of the time, according to the surgeons' own literature.

This surgery, which is often suggested by ophthalmologists, attempts to fix the eye by cutting muscle and then reattaching it in order to reposition the eye. However, since the brain was not in on this decision, the inner conditioning which is almost always responsible for the outer defect has not changed, and the operation frequently fails to straighten the eye. Repeated surgery is not unusual. Of course in some cases surgery may be necessary, but it should always be considered the treatment of last resort.

In neurology, research was demonstrating that different areas of the brain are responsible for the integration of data from the various senses, and that the cells throughout the brain interact with varying degrees of sophistication. In simple matters, we react almost instantly—a knee jerk; when more complicated thought is involved, a person appears to withdraw into himself. He gets a faraway look in his eyes as he searches for comprehension.

Man's brain was also shown to have an organization based on his evolution up the primate scale: automatic body functions we accomplish without thought are controlled at the base level; motor movements at another and thinking in the brain's most recent acquisition, the cerebral cortex, an area that does not even exist in the lower animals.

The brain of a human being develops along similar lines in the womb. The lower levels get into place first. The thinking man's cortex is the last to be organized and the first to be affected by disease. This being so, it is possible to accept the idea that behavior is governed by this cortex, and that as the neural tissue varies, so will behavior. If inappropriate conditioning, malnutrition, injury or surgery interfere with those tissue connections, behavior will be affected.

If certain behavioral patterns are not acquired in the usual sequence, more advanced patterns may be damaged. To repair them, therapy may have to start at the base level, even though the task, such as creeping and crawling, may seem foolish to a 10-year-old. But action at the base level opens a path to the next level, and one proceeds on that basis. In vision therapy, body balancing skills, which are learned in the first few years of life, often must be rehearsed and perfected as a way of reaching the specific problem that is now interfering with eye/ body coordination.

Adults, however, won't be asked to crawl around, but may be given a visual task while teetering on a balance board. It won't get you into the circus, but it may open up your eyes so that you don't bump into doors or knock over a glass of red wine on your neighbor's new rug. The white one.

The concept that behavior reflects the neural organization of the brain has led to many diverse points of view and modes of treatment. There are those who believe that once the brain is organized, it is unchangeable. Others propose that some control of behavior can be developed through exercises. Two men in Philadelphia treat on the premise that the injured brain can be reprogrammed through exercises which stimulate different brain functions, beginning at the lower level and then moving up. These men, Glenn Doman, a physical therapist, and Dr. Carl Delacato, an educational psychologist, treat retarded, autistic or otherwise brain-damaged children who are usually considered beyond help.

Beginning at the beginning is also the basis for a relatively new method of treating autistic children, who show little connection to others, and may not even talk. Some consider autism a response to a lack of emotional warmth from the parents. The treatment: The child sits on his mother's lap and is simply held in her arms for 20 minutes a day, even though he may long be past the age where this is normal, say 10 or 12. In this situation it is hard for the parent and child to avoid looking each other in the eye, and it may be that the affection which develops between them, and later others, is deeply linked to his most basic cue—eye contact.

As stated earlier, certain life experiences, including learning visual skills, should occur at specific times when the gates are open and the system sensitive to specific experiences which lead to specific behavior. In other words, if A doesn't happen, B might not either. Learning how to live well requires that all the building blocks be put into the right place at the right time. Interference anywhere along the line is reflected in inappropriate behavior and also sets up a chain reaction.

While the world—the scientists at least—was assimilating this information, a research psychologist in France, Jean Piaget, came up with a theory of how we develop intellectually. With a biologist's background, he proposed that as concepts form, the brain is modified. Neuroanatomy today shows the brain undergoing tiny shifts of structural alteration as we absorb whatever the constantly changing environment has to offer. Tissue accommodates itself to the peculiarities of the event, whether it be an object or a concept.

After thousands of years, neurology combined with psychology was about to confirm an ancient theory which gives mind and body, genes and environment their separate but equal stature in the growth and development of intelligence and behavior. We had the information to focus our image of what a man is, how he got to be that way and how he must care for himself.

An eclectic mind synthesized the precepts in all of the above fields and postulated how vision is related to behavior and personality. A. M. Skeffington, an optometrist, developed a formula for examining all the skills involved in vision and perception, showing how these might be trainable to a certain degree. Later his wife, Mary Jane Skeffington, an ophthalmologist, continued his work.

Skeffington's premise was certainly not a new one, but a melding of many: Since vision is learned and occurs in the brain, to retrain (or recondition) that process we need to alter the environment, or the input. This could be done with a program of vision therapy that would guide what the eyes send to the visual cortex and eventually straighten out misperception. Then we could see better and understand more.

The procedures may seem like exercises for the eyes, but their impact is in the visual cortex where perception occurs. The eyes are the pathways; the exercises are the tools.

But theories need statistical proof to be acceptable. Other researchers, notably Meredith Morgan and Glenn Fry, in the next few decades would provide the academic underpinnings. By evaluating the responses of thousands of patients they determined what is normal, thereby providing a basis for deciding who needs therapy and who doesn't.

Unfortunately, although their work was well documented, it is still filtering down slowly to the average practitioner and the general public.

There have been theories of "sight without glasses" through eye exercises for decades, and although one, the Bates method, named for the physician who developed the program, found acceptance with some segments of the public and intrigued the medical profession, the methods were too imprecise, the claims too great, for it to be taken seriously.

The most famous advocate of the Bates method was Aldous Huxley, who wrote about his recovery from near blindness in *The Art of Seeing,* a book which has long been out of print, but due to a resurgence of interest in vision was recently re-issued in paperback.

Today Skeffington's work has been advanced by research at the

Gesell Institute of Child Development, the Optometric Center of New York, optometric colleges throughout the country and individual practitioners, just as in any branch of medicine many minds work both independently and together to further the scope of knowledge.

Behavioral optometry is still an emerging field, with only a few hundred specialists throughout the country. Almost all are optometrists, not opthalmologists, M.D.s whose training is basically in surgery and treating disease.

Traditional medicine shows a reluctance to even debate the issue, regardless of the statistics and research which demonstrate that something more than placing a highly polished lens in front of the eye is needed to be sure we are seeing everything.

How Vision Therapy Works

Getting your eyes examined should be more than an annual checkup to find out whether your lenses need to be strengthened or to pick out more stylish frames. While a behavioral optometrist may prescribe traditional corrective lenses, he begins with the premise that your vision can be protected from deteriorating, developed to its potential and enhanced to meet special needs.

Instead of simply looking for disease and testing for acuity, which means that you can read letters on a chart at 20 feet (which most people could also read at 20 feet on a chart devised in 1863), the vision therapist will check a wide variety of visual skills, some of which you may not even realize affect your general behavior and outlook. He will test your binocular skill (how well you use your eyes together), spatial judgement (knowing where objects are in space), accommodative abilities (shifting focus from far to near), visual memory (which helps your spelling), eye/body and eye/hand coordination (how well you can dance the foxtrot or hustle, or how legible your handwriting is), visualization (practicing in your mind's eye how to act in a particular situation), and perceptual flexibility (the ability to empathize with another's point of view).

Along with a complete medical record he will ask you to give a personality sketch of yourself. How you walk, talk and what you say —in short, your demeanor and outlook on life—will be considered, along with the demands your occupation makes on your eyes, and if your visual skills are commensurate with your age and needs. An accountant's needs are vastly different from a forest ranger's. A behavioral optometrist will try to determine if your occupation and habits are putting your eyes under undue stress, and may prescribe preventive lenses to alleviate the strain and keep your vision from deteriorating. That way, when you take off your glasses, your eyes have a better chance of being at least as good as when you put them on; preventive lenses nip the problem in the bud, before it dims the vision.

You may do remarkably well reading those letters on the chart, but good vision includes all those other skills, and more. Vision is tied up with how a person moves, thinks, comes to a decision; visual problems can give us clues to what kinds of stresses the person operates under. Distortions of the eye are considered to be problems in reaching a decision, reflections of behavioral style, and indications of some form of stress, whether it be physiological, cultural or environmental. It just might be something as simple as the fact that you didn't have proper lighting on the bedside table all those nights you stayed up until three o'clock and secretly read while your parents thought you were sleeping.

As vision changes, so may personality and behavior. This was the case of a 13-year-old who wore thick glasses, was slow in school and extremely reticent and shy. Many of the academic problems which plagued Brigitte for years might have been avoided if her wandering eye had been corrected when she was young. When Brigitte arrived from Sweden last year to live with her aunt and uncle in Manhattan, her aunt thought she had a sweet but dull girl on her hands—someone who read almost not at all. After five minutes of studying, she would rearrange her shelves or daydream. She was uncoordinated and played almost no sports. Headaches plagued her almost daily. She had asked the school nurse for aspirin so often that the nurse began refusing her, convinced that either something was drastically wrong or the child was using this ploy to get attention.

The aunt became aware that one of Brigitte's eyes wandered rather than looking straight and sharp. She questioned the opthalmologist during a regular examination to check Brigitte's prescription for nearsightedness, and he said it would probably clear up by itself.

Brigitte's aunt was not pleased with the answer, and mentioned it to an optometrist. She wondered what could be done if Brigitte ever wanted to wear contacts. Although not a vision therapist himself, he was familiar with the work and suggested that Brigitte be tested by one.

The examination revealed that Brigitte's two eyes weren't working together, and the wandering eye was seeing hardly at all. Brigitte's shyness and fear of seeming to be a problem to her American family kept her from telling the doctor about her headaches, but the doctor figured that she was likely to be troubled with them, and frequently.

"Do you get headaches?" he asked. "Oh, sometimes," she said in a voice barely above a whisper. "How often? Two or three times a day?" "Yes, that's right. Doesn't everybody? When they read?"

Because her problems were acute, and her low grades were keeping her out of a better school ("She's not our type of student," the aunt was told), an intensive program of therapy was begun. Brigitte had exercises to do at home and came to the office twice a week. At the end of three months, her grades shot up into the 90's. The headaches? What headaches? They had stopped weeks earlier. Brigitte not only reads what she has to for school, she now reads for her own enjoyment. Before, she wouldn't even bother leafing through *Seventeen*. She's become more outgoing and is planning to learn tennis, which she'd tried and failed at before. And last fall she entered a good private school. She had become their "type of student."

The exercises and procedures in vision therapy are designed to teach a person to use his nerve and muscle systems better and put them at the command of the mind. The aim is not just the ability to see in the laboratory but to make the eyes work well in everyday life, with all its uncertainties, distractions and disappointments.

What occurs at a behavioral optometrist's office at first appears to be child's play: putting pegs into holes on a revolving turntable; standing in front of a blackboard drawing circles with each hand at the same time; looking through a gadget and tracing a simple picture; playing with pieces of plastic—triangles, rectangles, squares—and putting them together to form certain shapes; standing on a teetering balance board while staring at a multicolored revolving disc; looking at 3–D pictures and shifting focus from one point that appears close to one that seems far away; wearing thick training lenses to create an extra blur and trying to pick out random letters on a ball swinging at the end of a cord; pointing to numbers on a chart to the beat of a metronome; the program is tailored to the individual's needs, and most specialists work with several patients at a time as each does different exercises.

Individual therapy is suggested for children who are not able to work in a group, or for adults who require an intimate interaction to help them deal with their new perceptions.

The tasks may sound uncomplicated, but they're not for the person with impaired vision. Depending on the gravity of the vision problems, the skills will come more or less slowly. Then there is the way a person feels about what he is doing. A patient coming to grips with the fact that he has been seeing in a way which limits perception will come to comprehend he does this in other areas of his life, and suddenly a wealth of behavioral information comes springing forth.

Co-author Lorraine Dusky (henceforth referred to as L.D.), who was once a patient of Richard Kavner (R.K.), explains her reaction this way:

In the beginning, except for the fact that one of my eyes was severely nearsighted, I wasn't aware that I had other vision problems. I knew I bumped into things frequently but didn't think this had anything to do with my sight.

A few months after therapy began I was doing exercises which were designed to make both eyes work together. I was looking at aerial photographs of Paris through a stereoscope. The task was to make a single image out of the two I was seeing. We had been at this for weeks, and frankly I was tired and frustrated that I wasn't getting anyplace.

Then all of a sudden—one image! Immediately I got hot flashes in the brain, and I knew something strange and uncomfortable was going on up there.

I can't really verbalize how I sensed that something was amiss up in the gray matter, but the feeling was strong. My stomach got upset—I thought I would throw up. My eyes teared and my head ached.

I knew that I wanted to see differently, if only to see a single image of the Eiffel Tower, but I knew that a lot of other changes were accompanying this one. I sensed that it wasn't just in my vision that I was confined—that my outlook had been narrow, and this touched every aspect of my life. I suddenly realized I didn't like the way my life had been going, and I didn't know quite what to do about it. I wanted to let go, but aye, there's the rub, I was afraid to because I didn't know what it would be like out there. What's unknown is always scary.

I calmed down in a few minutes, and the physical symptoms passed. R.K. had me try the picture again. I got one image. Again. And again. And again.

When I left the office that day, I called three friends until I got one who could have a martini lunch with me. I ordinarily talk a lot anyway, but this day I felt a bit as if I were coming apart and had to find some safe ground to get glued back together. Eventually, instead of boring my friends with all my self-discoveries, I went into therapy with a psychiatrist.

When did this narrow perspective start, I wondered. I phoned my mother and asked if I had spent a lot of time confined in the playpen. (I didn't phrase the question quite that way.) Yes, she said, adding that I had not crawled much, but went straight to walking—only I had tried to run first and fell on my face for quite a while. I was so intent on getting out of the playpen and moving that I didn't want to have to do it slowly. Naturally, I didn't learn to walk until I learned how to slow down. I still walk quickly.

She also told me that when I was young I was constantly bumping into doors and other stationary objects. When she asked a doctor if anything was wrong with my eyes, he told her not to worry, the problem would clear up by itself.

Through therapy I was beginning to learn how to use my two eyes together and get a better control over my environment. I didn't have to continue to bump into objects, or go whizzing through life as if I had roller skates permanently attached to my feet.

The period of disorientation described above is called *critical empathy.* Some patients break down completely, sobbing and crying. Such reactions are akin to those which occur during other types of psychotherapy—notably primal scream. In that type of therapy a person unlocks his feelings and old memories, and in doing so is conscious of pain and discomfort as he lets the bad feelings go. The resolution of those feelings is necessary to reduce the physiological stress.

While such violent reactions to vision therapy may seem extreme, Lawrence MacDonald of the Massachusetts College of Optometry finds them not unusual—when it is accepted that for every emotional problem the patient has locked his feelings and memories into a particular family of muscles, and this often occurs in the muscles of the eyes. The Reichians call this *armoring.*

"Every so-called neurotic problem involves the functioning of the total organism," MacDonald states. "What appears to be a minor modification of visual habits may in fact have deeper underlying implications in terms of total behavior. It is probably true that visual problems also involve emotional problems, and many emotional problems also involve visual problems."

Some, including Dr. MacDonald, believe that critical empathy constitutes a breakthrough for the patient, who afterward is able to reorganize his visual world and attain those abilities which had previously eluded him. At times it is not necessary to push the patient to such an extreme level, but better to stop a particular exercise for the time being, when physical discomfort sets in. That way the patient is not left at loose ends with an emotional storm he doesn't know how to handle. Slowly removing the patient's resistance to a new way of seeing lets him put his own psychological building blocks into place.

These intense, vivid reactions to changes in perception do not occur in everybody. Children almost never experience them, probably because they do not have as much time and emotion invested in continuing their misperception.

Vision therapy is sometimes more effective when combined with other types of therapy, including psychoanalysis or one of the body therapies. This may help the individual find some way of dealing with the blocked emotions that come rushing out. Sometimes making a person aware of the psychological reaction to a visual problem is enough to enable him to make a change by himself. At other times he needs help.

An inappropriate emotional response or behavior ingrained over a long period of time can frequently be reached only through a psychological approach. Sometimes changes in vision cause the psychological changes. And at other times psychological changes cause visual changes. A nearsighted person, for instance, may start thinking in broader terms when his vision improves. Or the vision may change but the person can't act upon it to carry it over into other areas of his life. All that is known for sure is that when vision changes, it is not the eye alone that changes.

Of course, vision therapy is not an alternative to psychotherapy. Vision therapy is for visual problems only. If it eliminates a psychological problem as a by-product of treatment, well and good. Unfortunately, some psychological problems persist and require other types of therapy.

Although the premise that vision has a marked effect on personality has not yet infiltrated traditional schools of psychotherapy, a small number of psychiatrists and psychologists are beginning to recognize the research. New York City psychotherapist Dr. Garnet Beach suggests to many of her patients that they be tested for vision problems. In her work with children, Dr. Beach estimates that a full 50 percent of their emotional disturbances are rooted in visual impairments, mostly correctable. Children may respond quicker to vision therapy than adults because the problem has not been entrenched for so long a time, but this is not always the case. Motivation is the key factor, not age.

According to Dr. Beach, "One of the ways we develop our comprehension of what is real and what is not, of what we will have to do in order to survive, is through our perceptual cues—smell, touch, hearing, taste and sight—and when there is a misfiring along the way, we deprive ourselves of information that we need to operate efficiently. Any arresting of information hinders us in some way."

Dr. Beach became conscious of the eye-and-mind relationship when she observed that the cause of a significant number of the problems of disturbed children who had had complete physical and psychological work-ups appeared to be neither entirely organic nor entirely emotional, but somewhere in the middle. "And I had the feeling that all these youngsters looked at me strangely," she says. "There was a vagueness there, a lack of focus—people call it *soft eyes.*"

Eventually she sent a hyperactive child, a nonreader, to be tested. The eight-year-old had already had her eyes examined three times before, and her acuity was good. Her parents, both psychologists, were told that the problem was not in her sight. This time, however, an extensive examination showed that the child was not coordinating her eyes. As a result of vision therapy she was able to learn how to read. She is now reading at her grade level in school and doing well.

The young man with the severe crossed eyes mentioned earlier responded when psychotherapy was accompanied by vision therapy. For several years he had been in orthoptic therapy alone, and while he reported that his strabismus was alleviated somewhat, it would eventually return. The psychotherapy in his past had been unfruitful. Only when the two therapies were undertaken together was there lasting improvement.

Because visual symptoms sometimes are the way we adapt to psychological stress, giving up the crutch can be painful. "We've had less information and consequently fewer choices. And letting go of that old way gives a person an empty feeling for a while," Dr. Beach adds.

The reason that vision—more than the other senses—plays such a crucial role in shaping personality is because in man the visual sense dominates. It is the way we receive between 80 to 90 percent of our information about the world. It is the reason film is such a valuable teaching aid.

That people instinctively understand this is reflected in a 1976 Gallup poll about what people feel is the worst thing that could happen to them: Blindness was second on the list, outranked only by cancer.

None of this has ever troubled lovers. They have always known that the eyes are the mirror of the mind. "Eyes without speaking confess the secrets of the heart," St. Jerome wrote centuries ago. It appears that he may have turned out to be a farsighted prophet.

2
How You See Is Who You Are

It lies in the nature of a strong man to press forward. In so doing he encounters obstructions. Therefore he returns to the way suited to his situation, where he is free to advance or to retreat.

Anything from the joy of receiving a letter from a lover to the uncertainty of crossing a busy intersection activates the body's mechanisms to some degree, because that is how we adapt to the changing circumstances of life.

Emotional responses and their physical counterparts can be either helpful or harmful to our health and well-being, according to biologist Dr. Hans Selye, whose work shows us that stress is an integral part of our lives. Although we are not sure which came first, the state of mind or the behavior, we do know they generally operate as a matched set. Each physical or biological action causes a psychological response of some sort, and vice versa.

When the response to the stress is inappropriate and we do not adapt easily, we may get ourselves into all kinds of trouble: high blood pressure, allergies, ulcers, certain types of rheumatic, cardiovascular and renal diseases and emotional disturbances. Selye contends that these ailments appear to be essentially diseases of adaptation.

To the list we would add the myriad eye problems afflicting literate man in the last half of the twentieth century. Our eyes have not adapted themselves to the environment.

Change rarely comes easily; what is necessary is to decide if it is worth the price and then proceed one way or the other. Not making a decision is one in itself, for the lives and circumstances of others will proceed or regress, and the effects they produce will in turn affect our lives. Seemingly, all that will have happened is that others will have

30

made the choices for us. But there's always the flash of awareness of what might have been. The point is: changes on the outside cause changes on the inside. Environment affects the body.

As long as we can handle stress and return to normal without a great deal of fuss, we are healthy; however, if we get stuck in the stress-response pattern and are unable to shift back to relaxation, the stress will ultimately overtax us and result in illness.

The eyes in particular have a critical stake in our psychological/physiological makeup, since connections from the eyes to the brain are so numerous. The brain receives more sensory stimulation from the eyes than it does from any of our other senses. In the approach to vision which considers our eyes outposts of the brain, the biology and psychology of a person cannot be separated. We realize this concept represents a new and different way of thinking about eyes and vision, as far as most people are concerned. However, the evidence here was not dreamed up by a mad scientist sitting in a room and pondering Life. It is the result of data collected methodically for decades.

Numerous studies have documented that people with similar types of visual problems often share similar personality characteristics. In fact, one psychological survey was able to detect more than three-quarters of the nearsighted children who participated. Such a finding indicates it might be possible to determine those who might become myopic and suggest ways to avoid it.

Changing visual habits does not mean you will acquire a new personality the way you buy a new suit of clothes. However, sometimes it may. A person's perception is often a mirror image of his attitude and behavior. For instance, if your friends continually refuse to ride in the car you drive you are likely to suspect there is more about you they don't like than your driving and react accordingly.

But once they start leaving the driving to you and sit back to offer companionship and conversation, isn't it likely you might respond with a more outgoing, convivial demeanor? Which is what happened to a tax attorney in her mid-fifties. When she first came to be examined, she was tense and highly critical of everything. Her rigid, taut attitude was noticed by the receptionist, who called the doctor's attention to her as she sat in the waiting room, bolt upright on the edge of her chair, pinched eyebrows frowning at the tropical fish, who didn't seem bothered by her in the least.

It turned out that her nearsightedness was being exacerbated by the failing sight all of us experience with age. Her bifocal prescription was getting stronger, and she couldn't function without her glasses. She felt chained to them—and she didn't like that at all.

When she began vision therapy, she fought every step of the way. If an exercise was difficult, *why was he doing this to her?* Any humorous comment was taken as a personal insult.

After a year of work her vision had improved to the point where she would go without her hated reading glasses. She was able to laugh at herself. The tightness in her face was gone, and she said that many of her friends remarked that her whole outlook had changed. What had she done? they asked. She simply smiled. *Nothing,* she said. *I haven't been to Elizabeth Arden.* And after her summer vacation, she delightedly reported that for the first time her companions would ride in her car. She said her driving had always made them nervous.

The changes in behavior will always be more subtle than the visual changes which can be measured in a doctor's office. A person in whom a particular way of acting and reacting has been ingrained for decades does not wake up one morning and find that the old patterns have dissipated with dreams. It does not matter whether our behavior patterns were put there by heredity or environment or both; they are part of us, and they stay, more or less, for the long haul. However, if we don't like something about ourselves, if our responses make us or our loved ones unhappy, we can try to change. That is what therapy—any variety—is all about.

Vision therapy is a process of learning how to change inappropriate visual habits to ones more compatible with a smooth and easy life. In doing so, inappropriate behavior often changes too. But the pattern may be so imbedded it is difficult to give up, even though the circumstances which initiated it have become ancient history.

Stress is the prime factor in setting the wheels in motion. When the demands are above and beyond what our eyes can handle, something has to give. Stress comes in two forms: physical trauma, which includes everything from dim lighting and illness to inadequate nutrition in the womb and a misshapen cranium at birth; and psychological trauma, from the death of a parent to academic work beyond one's ability. The psychological problem may be displaced to the eye, as well as possibly getting locked into other muscles, and the emotional response—fear, anger, loneliness—becomes connected with the visual one, each continually aiding and abetting the other.

We can react to trauma in two ways: fight or flight. Consider the pressure to achieve in school, which involves a great deal of reading. One survey found that the average college student reads 51 books a year. If you choose to wade through all of them, to *fight,* to push past the pain of tired eyes, your eyes eventually look for some way to accommodate you. Nearsightedness is one response, because they have adapted to seeing best only up close. On the other hand, if you choose *flight,* try to avoid the situation completely, you may become a nonreader or one who reads little and with difficulty. Many of this group are called dyslexic.

Both symptoms are occurring at a predictable rate in our schools. The amount and degree of myopia rises with the grades, and depending on who's calling it, estimates of dyslexia vary from 2 to 15 percent of all school children. Our data—and that of certain educators and child psychologists—suggest this need not be so. Obviously, this is not a call to shut down the schools but an attempt to have parents and educators think about what we are doing in our traditional halls of learning, albeit inadvertently: causing visual havoc.

The Hidden Problems

Approximately 70 percent of us have visual problems of which we are not even aware. Since most eye examinations do not check for these hidden problems, they go unrecognized. They include erratic eye tracking, sluggish or inefficient focusing, unstable fusion—eye-teaming skills, reduced peripheral awareness, insufficient depth perception and awkward eye/body and eye/hand coordination.

But instead of realizing that the trouble stems from our eyes, we end up at the doctor's or therapist's complaining of aches and pains without causes we can discern. Tiredness, lethargy, tension, irritability, anger, rigidity—all can be symptoms of visual problems. Inefficiency in the eyes can go a long way in playing havoc with our moods and bodies.

If we still lived free in the wilds, our eyes probably wouldn't run into the kinds of trouble they do today when we require them to take on tasks for which they are not biologically prepared. It's like asking someone who's never run a mile to try out for the Olympic team. Our eyes valiantly try to go the distance but may fade in the stretch and break down. It doesn't always put us in eyeglasses or become as obvious as a crossed eye, but it does cause confusion on the subconscious level and often leads to those vague aches and pains, or fatigue at the end of the day which puts you in bed as soon as you walk in the door. Those who listen to their bodies will quit before the spine is permanently curved or the ulcer is festering or the migraine has galloped in for a stay; but not all listen well, or at all. This generation's training has been to prize the mighty intellect and to reward the indefatigable student.

To understand the breakdowns, we must understand the eyes' miraculous abilities and how stress affects them: *Eye-tracking* problems concern the ability to locate an object and follow it smoothly through space. If you can't do that efficiently—and you won't necessarily know if you can't—you will skip words as you read, find yourself rereading lines and phrases to pick up the words you missed, read slower than you would otherwise have to, and you may use a finger or a marker to guide your eyes across the page. You'll think you're not too bright, and so will others around you.

Any sport requiring you to follow a small object and react will be difficult: tennis, basketball, baseball. When driving, you'll be the sort who hesitates at the crossroads and when changing lanes. You know you aren't an accurate judge of how long it will take the oncoming car to reach you. The guy honking his horn behind you just increases the tension.

One test to determine who is schizophrenic and who is not is based on the individual's ability to track a ball swinging at the end of a string. The inability to aim precisely and know where things are in space is considered by some to be a clue to schizophrenia and can be used to indicate who else in the family is susceptible. While schizophrenics are probably going to do poorly at the test, of course not all people who fail are schizophrenic, or likely to become so.

Focusing or *accommodation* gives us the detail, separating the figure from the background, and because it is related to reading and putting objects into categories, appears to be closely connected with intellect. Focusing is the ability to adjust the eyes to know WHAT something is.

People who have such problems will have trouble seeing the difference between *e* and *o, these* and *those.* Fuzzy focusers frequently do not have good language skills, but, surprisingly, some of them turn up in occupations such as editor, in which the sustained ability to focus for long periods of time is a necessity. The person who chooses to fight on through the discomfort may end up with a physical problem, or simply be one highly irritable editor by mid-afternoon.

Possible signals that focusing is the problem include unusual fatigue or restlessness when concentrating on a target, finding that letters and lines run together or jump around, seeing a blur when reading or writing and holding reading matter excessively close.

Focusing usually develops at approximately three months, and mom is the usual target. But if she feels uncomfortable with the baby's gaze and doesn't meet it with hers, the child may not learn to focus properly and later have difficulty showing affection, for the gaze is the way we communicate this message to one another wordlessly. If somebody has shifty eyes, he's hard to trust or to love. If a person avoids your gaze, it is frequently seen as a signal that the news is bad or the truth it isn't, while in fact it may just be a habit stemming from early experiences.

The problem may also be a biochemical one, for focusing is a function of the smooth muscle system. If this isn't operating up to snuff, the faulty focusing may be just one of several related smooth-muscle problems: allergies, irregular bowel movements, indigestion, upper respiratory infections such as colds and a high histamine level, which means you are prone to allergies. The smooth muscles are controlled by the involuntary system which regulates the glands which in turn control the body's functions.

Integration between aiming and focusing skills keeps them—and us—in a happy balance. Aiming tells us WHERE something is; focusing gives the brain a clear image so we can see what it is, and if the two aren't on a friendly basis and operating smoothly together, the result is a combination of the difficulties outlined above.

Aiming is controlled by the voluntary muscles—you want to look east, you look east. Focusing is directed by the involuntary system. Your eyes focus automatically on your golden retriever as he sneaks out through a hole in the hedge to go gallivanting around the neighborhood.

At approximately age one these two systems link up and form a brotherly bond, but it's necessary for each to allow the other a certain bit of freedom. Not too little, not too much. Think of these systems as gears in traction: one starts up, the other follows suit. But there needs to be a certain amount of leeway between the two.

If the linkage is too loose and sloppy, one system is way ahead of the other, and the person experiences some difficulty in integrating where his eyes are looking and what he sees. He is likely to be loose and disorganized in his thinking and acting, and sometimes just can't seem to get things together.

Conversely, if the gears are too tightly jammed together, one interferes with the smooth functioning of the other, and causes friction and discomfort. Each skill needs an almost imperceptible amount of time to make adjustments freely without interference from the other, but if they are too tightly bound, each has trouble. People with this problem will often avoid doing close work, or become irritable when they do. You probably won't get many letters from this type of person—even if he protests his love for you on the telephone—and have you ever met anyone whose irritability rises with the amount and length of concentration required for the task? Say the wrong word and Bang!

Both types will usually have a combination of the reading difficulties mentioned under focusing and aiming.

Binocular fusion is the ability to use both eyes together well, to team them up so that they complement each other rather than compete to give us one clear picture with depth. Convergence tells a person where something is in relation to him. At its most serious level, a fusion problem results in a crossed eye, but a great many people have insufficiencies that aren't so apparent. When a large group is examined for binocular skills, a full 70 percent are found to have a deficiency.

The skill begins developing at six months. For the next several years an individual practices it and should come to age six with the skill operating smoothly. If not, something is obviously happening along the way. Although the problem may have a physiological or psychological underpinning, it is more likely the result of not developing to the level of sophistication we demand today. The degree of proficiency which develops normally may be adequate for that farmer we keep talking about: evolutionary readiness is always an adaptation to what has gone before. After all, it is improbable that such a large majority would have such a gross defect built in. The statistics attest to the fact that *we have old eyes in a new age.*

When a person has poor binocular skills, he is under constant stress to maintain a balance of some sort to keep from becoming worse. Such an individual is like someone on the verge of a breakdown—but fighting every step of the way to maintain equilibrium. It takes a lot of energy. He probably rubs his eyes frequently, rests his head on his arm when writing, trying to block one eye out, sits awkwardly when reading or writing, has poor eye/hand coordination and sporadic double vision. The binocular skills give our images depth, and without that last refinement it is hard to understand where objects are in space.

Without good depth perception, a person has difficulty catching a

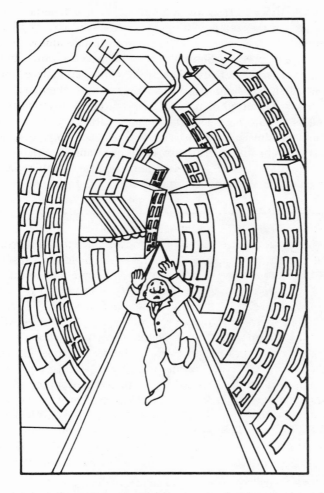

A person with inadequate depth perception may feel that the world is closing in on him.

ball, feels quite queasy walking over a bridge or standing at the edge of a terrace, and probably doesn't enjoy window tables in restaurants high in the sky, for he is always uncertain of where he is in relation to the edge. Given a choice, he'll take an apartment on the third floor rather than the tenth. He may tell himself intellectually he's not going to fall out of the window, but he somehow doesn't feel it in his bones. He needs to hold onto a railing when going down steps because he is uneasy about the space in front of him and has difficulty judging precisely where the edge of the step is.

In crowds he feels extremely uncomfortable because he feels people are closing in on him. Shopping a week before Christmas will put him into a panic—and not just because he can't get waited on quickly. This feeling of spatial suffocation can come and go, because when he is sick, run down, depressed or upset, he cannot compensate for the problem as well as he can when he is happy and healthy.

His handwriting is likely to be crooked or poorly spaced, and while he may do all right in algebra because he can think problems through, geometry is another matter, since to comprehend it, he must understand relationships of form, or how edges in space relate to one another.

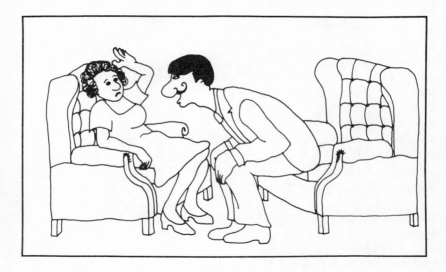

A man with excessive convergence meets someone with the opposite problem: His need for proximity violates her need for distance.

The problem can be generally of two types. If an individual has convergence insufficiency (which means he has difficulty coordinating and concentrating on objects and people close at hand) he typically is going to want to maintain a personal distance. He will stand back when talking to others and feel uncomfortable or threatened when someone closes in on him. He'd rather talk to three people than to one, because that keeps him distant from any one in particular. If he's also farsighted, this attitude will be more marked, and he may avoid close personal relationships.

In contrast, someone with too much convergence tends to move in close. He will not only stand near but seek relationships which are extremely intimate (especially if he's nearsighted)—and drive the person with the opposite problem right up the wall. One moves in and the other backs away. The marriage maven says: not a good bet.

Perceptual skills allow us to make use of the abilities of our eyes. It is how we put the information together in the brain and comprehend what we see. Once the information comes into the visual centers in the brain, it goes to memory, it goes to language, and somewhere along the line it is sorted out from all the other data. The mind exclaims *Aha!* and we understand. The problem in perception can surface as either a difficulty in categorizing objects (form perception) or in understanding the relationship of one thing to another (spatial perception).

People with difficulty in perceiving forms have trouble fitting objects into categories, for they cannot easily comprehend how something is similar or dissimilar in relation to something else. Their minds are like post offices lacking neatly defined cubbyholes for each district and size of package; instead, there is a large cubbyhole over here, a tiny one over there. It's difficult to sort the mail. Once they do label something, they have trouble changing its category, for they will cling to one —at least they have labeled it. They may be overly specific and not see the forest for the trees, or not be able to discern that the two are different categories of the same thing; or be overly general and claim, for instance, that all women drive the same way.

When reading they will mistake words with the same or similar beginnings, fail to recognize the same word in the next sentence or the next book. They may make errors copying from reference materials to a notebook and confuse objects which have only minor differences.

Fitting the pieces together escapes these people and their approach to life is somewhat disorganized—and their homes and offices are probably messy, too. Rather than structure, they go on intuition.

In the last few years neurology has given us an understanding of the brain's architecture indicating that it is split into two hemispheres, right and left, and each side governs different aspects of personality and behavior, with one hemisphere dominating. The left side is a whiz at languages, logic and the mechanics of things; while the right brain governs emotion, matters creative and psychic, and intuition. In each person, one side may dominate, so that it could be that an individual with such a problem is ruled by the right brain.

They will have trouble with road maps, and when they direct their own body through space will often bump into things, perhaps even walk in a crooked line. In language, metaphors and similes escape them, and they do not do well on analogy tests for they simply do not see how a picture or a word is like or unlike the others in the series.

Because they have poor judgement of space and time, they are the people who are almost always late—and arrive full of apologies. You see, they thought they had allowed enough time to get across town, but the bus didn't come the minute they stepped out the door, or the traffic was terrible! It does no good to point out that five o'clock traffic in midtown is always terrible.

Nearsightedness or Myopia

Nearsightedness is on the rise. While that blunt statement may only elicit a *So what else is new?* reaction, consider what it means in terms of our culture: we are becoming a generation of handicapped persons. It is not unlikely that if you are reading this book you already own a pair of glasses for myopia. The age at which it is beginning is going down from adolescence to the pre-school years, and the number it affects keeps going up, especially among the highly educated. It is estimated that a full 25 percent of our population is nearsighted, while among other peoples of the world, the tendency is to be what we call farsighted. If myopia is inherited, from whom did we inherit it?

Yet traditional medicine clings to the idea that myopia is caused by an inherited elongation of the eyeball, and furthermore that there is nothing we can do except resort to stronger and stronger glasses. But what caused the eyeball to lengthen? Why weren't our forefathers nearsighted to the same degree that we are? Nearsightedness is practically unknown where book learning is not prized. In our culture city-bred folk are more prone to myopia than their country cousins. Honor students and graduate students have higher degrees of myopia than school dropouts.

If myopia were simply a condition which happened to some and didn't happen to others, these statistical variables would not follow this orderly and predictable pattern:

• Before age 10 approximately four to six percent of the population is nearsighted. By the time children are through the eighth grade, 20 percent are nearsighted. At the end of high school the number has jumped to 40 percent. And throughout college the number varies from 60 to 80 percent, with the higher percentages among the honors and graduate students. No other sense is prone to such an overwhelming amount of illness, which, in effect, is what nearsightedness is.

• At the U.S. Naval Academy the first-year plebes arrive with good acuity, since it is a requirement for admission. By graduation, a high percentage have become myopic. In one class more than half ended up nearsighted.

• A study at Dartmouth found that those with the most severe eye defects were the best achievers. At Harvard the amount of myopia increased for each year spent in graduate school.

• Among children of migrant workers, who are never in school for any great length of time, the incidence of myopia remains a fairly constant 6 percent. Farm children, who are likely to spend more time outdoors than their city cousins, gazing restfully at the horizon, have less myopia than city kids.

• In a survey of Eskimo families only two out of 130 children who could not read or write showed myopia; yet among their children who were attending school and eating a Western diet, at least at lunchtime, approximately 65 percent were nearsighted. This happened in a single generation in a population known to be somewhat farsighted. When the grandparents were examined, they showed the same lack of myopia as their children, the parents of the nearsighted group. If vision is truly inherited, the grandchildren should be farsighted—but they were nearsighted. Yet most of us still cling to the false assumption that nearsightedness is inherited if it tends to run in families, although this example shows massive reversal in a single generation. Genetics certainly cannot account for it.

Dr. Francis Young, a psychologist at Washington State University, makes an analogy to illustrate the illogical thinking here: if an English-speaking person marries an English-speaking person, they will give birth to an infant who also becomes an English-speaking person. But is the English inherited?

Dr. Young's extensive animal studies with monkeys and chimpanzees demonstrated that myopia can be induced in these primate cousins of ours under conditions not unlike those we frequently put ourselves through: dim lighting and limited visual field. Remember, the alert eye at rest is gazing off into the distance.

Which brings us back to Eskimos. Once they learned how to read and books were available, they went at it full blast. Possibly because there aren't that many other things to do during the long winter night, which goes on for months unrelieved by daylight above the Arctic Circle. In addition, the electric lighting in Eskimo homes is dim—usually a single 40 or 60 watt bulb in a room 10 feet by 10 feet or so. The conditions couldn't be better to encourage myopia. Our own youngsters show a similar relationship between studying and myopia, with a greater percentage of myopia during the school year than when examined at the end of summer, a time of few books and long hours outdoors. Yet few doctors take this into consideration, prescribing glasses at the end of the school year, unaware that the condition might improve during the vacation. The end result is that a crutch is given to a weak eye that might have gotten better on its own. With the crutch, the eye stays in its myopic state until it is permanently nearsighted.

In Japan, before World War II, the figures for myopia did not differ markedly from those for the United States. During the difficult years of the war, education was neglected; when the fighting stopped and schools were about to resume, it was discovered that myopia among the student population had halved. While a full 60 percent of the university students were nearsighted before the war, only 30 percent of the college-age population was at the end of the war. As the years went by and education continued, the incidence of myopia rose. The Japanese are back to their pre-war figures.

We could go on with studies and statistics, but they all tell the same story: as literacy rises, so does myopia. And yet books continue to be written stating that myopia is probably inherited—the result of a lengthening of the eyeball, causing the focus to shift from the surface of the retina to a spot in front of it. But why did the eyeball stretch out?

Genetics? The Eskimo study alone would seem to disprove a hereditary factor. It appears that something we are doing to ourselves causes the rapid increase of myopia. It is true that nearsighted parents will often have children who become nearsighted, but this likely results from certain personality traits: ambition, inhibition, scholarliness.

An eight-year study initiated at the Gesell Institute of Child Development showed that the amount of myopia expected in a group of upper middle class children (meaning well educated) could be dramatically reduced. The method: bringing lighting up to optimal conditions, making architectural modifications, replacing some book learning with physical activities combining feeling with seeing and also providing an opportunity for problem-solving. For instance, a child might be asked to determine the size of a room without a yardstick. Instead of answering the problem in feet or meters, a room might be so many of the child's footsteps long and so many wide.

The Gesell Institute's system was tried out in the Cheshire School district in Connecticut where a full 20 percent of the children could be expected to have myopia by the time they are in the sixth grade. Yet by relieving some of the continued strain of near-point work, that number has been halved, according to John Streff, who headed the program. Among the girls myopia was reduced by two-thirds. Girls usually have more myopia and at a younger age than boys, probably because females try harder to please and are thus likely to spend more time studying than males, who would just as soon play football.

The Chinese, a population long noted for seriousness—and a high degree of myopia—have put into practice what we should already know. The result has been a decrease in myopia, according to their own journals. In addition to routine calisthenics, students do eye exercises in class for 10 minutes twice a day. So do most factory workers. Glasses, although they are readily available, are only infrequently seen on students and young factory workers who do close work, reports an optometrist who visited the mainland in 1976. There is even an official poster of eye exercises.

If the percentages of myopia can be manipulated so handily, is it not logical to assume that we are doing something to cause it? The critical factor always comes down to one thing: long periods of unrelieved focus at near-point. Reading. Writing. Arithmetic. Those very things which our culture prizes above all else. Throw in several hours of television daily. The focus might not be as close, but it's certainly not the same as running around outside.

To see clearly at near-point, eye muscles strain to bring the focus together on the retina. Kept up for a long time, the muscles find a way to accommodate themselves to the job: they get locked into place. But then they lose the ability to loosen up when you want to look far afield—off into the distance—which is what the eye is more suited for. *Distance vision is relaxed vision.*

In fact, there is some research which tentatively suggests that the amount of refractive error—or degree of myopia—measurable with a retinoscope can be somewhat changed by techniques to increase stress or induce relaxation in the patient. However, this work has not been done on any large scale.

In practice, measurements of myopia in patients undergoing vision therapy will sometimes rise as the degree of fretfulness or anxiety increases. L.D.'s myopia in her left eye, which was 20/200 when she began therapy, has been testing in the morning of a good day at 20/40; after a tiring day of near-point work, it shoots up to 20/60 or 20/70. And once she is aware that she's not doing well in an examination, she tries all the harder, increasing stress and further reducing acuity.

One young man who wanted to be a policeman was hindered by a small amount of myopia. His acuity was 20/40 without glasses; to enter the police academy it had to be 20/20. He called the doctor and explained that he had already flunked the examination once. He was planning to take the next one two weeks later. R.K. told him to change the date to four months later and come in three times a week. He was given glasses to make his eyes relax, which helped him to release the tightness holding the focus close.

By the time the four months had passed his acuity was 20/15 in one eye, 20/20 in the other, except when he was tense and anxious. Since that is what he was likely to be when he took the examination, he was told to wear the training lenses the entire day before the time of the exam, to walk in casually, take a deep breath and think, *What the hell . . .*

He is now one of New York City's finest.

Myopia does not happen overnight; it comes on slowly and may go unnoticed until a student complains that he can't see the blackboard or that his eyes tire easily. As we have explained, it appears to be caused by overworking the muscle to focus at near-point, since the open eye at rest is made for distance viewing.

The eye under constant stress tries to send a warning sign: pain. *Hey, you—I'm tired. Won't you stop reading for a while? Don't you feel like blinking your eyes, or rubbing them? Are they burning? I'm just trying to talk to you, but you won't listen. . . .* Athletes are allowed to talk about the pain they experience; the diligent student simply presses on to the next page.

Eventually, the eye/brain grows accustomed to the strain, gives up sending pain messages, but grumbles a bit when asked to see afar. *Why do we need to bother with that? I can do this close work for you so well. . . .*

After a long period of reading, there will be a slight amount of blurring when shifting focus to a distant point. *What's this? You want to look at a sunset? Humph! Why are you making my life so hard? But if that's what you really want, you're the boss.*

If the close-point stress continues at the same rate—and the student marches right along reading, reading, reading—the focusing ability for distance weakens to the point where there is actually a loss of acuity that can be measured on one of those old-fashioned eye charts. *I tried to tell you I needed a rest, but what did I get from you? Another book. Okay, I'm getting used to the idea. Still don't like it. Couldn't you take up skateboarding rather than coin collecting?*

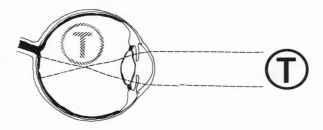

Myopia occurs when an image the eye receives comes to focus in front of the retina.

And as the near-point work continues, and the student works hard to stay on the honors list—he enjoys it—the eye muscles eventually lock into place; the pressure has been too great to resist. The eyeball lengthens and the image the eye receives comes to a focus in front of the retina, rather than on it, as in healthy vision. *Okay, you win. Now I've given you an eye perfectly suited to the life of a scholar. You know, the kind of shy, introverted kid who always has his nose buried in a book, doesn't go out much for sports and delights in showing off in the classroom. He doesn't do too well in sports anyway—he doesn't hit the basket or somehow he's not too coordinated. . . .*

Sounds like a string of cliches about the youngster who starts wearing glasses in the first grade? Well, the psychologists, psychiatrists and other researchers who study the matter say the cliches are more or less true. Generalizations, of course, but still statistically on the graph.

Such was the case of an extremely bright, shy, and pretty 10-year-old girl who came to the office a few years ago. She was soft-spoken to the point where she had to be asked to speak up so you could hear her. Her vision was 20/400, which meant her glasses were on the thick side. She wore them all the time, even when she took tap dancing and ballet lessons.

After a little over a year of therapy her acuity improved to 20/60;

she no longer needed glasses all of the time. Slowly the shyness fell away, and one day she asked if R.K. would like to see her tap dance. She put on her tap shoes and entertained everybody in the office. She's 13 now and headed for a career in the theater.

Naturally, not all myopes are going to take off their glasses and discover they are really Sarah Bernhardts. Most of them will pursue the interest that led them to become nearsighted in the first place: book learning. They will do it in school, in the library after school, at night at their desks, and when the lights are supposed to be out, they will read under the covers with a flashlight.

Behavior and personality studies on myopes and other visual types have been done since the early 1900s. Although they show a clustering of the same characteristics, they should not be taken as gospel for every individual—nor is a single person likely to exhibit all of the traits. With that in mind read on, and have fun reflecting on yourself and your friends.

Again and again, myopes have been found to be introverted, introspective, shy, meticulous (that attention to detail), disinclined to sports, and to have a marked preference for sedentary activities. They are self-centered, dogmatic, diligent, and in control of their emotions; they tend to be ambitious and pursue occupations which have high status in our culture: the professor versus the businessman, even if he is an executive. Probably due to their highly developed verbal skill, they are often leaders in social situations where talking is the key to success. Thus a myope might not dazzle on the dance floor, but can hold court on the sidelines, that is, if he's not too shy from lack of social experience.

In choosing an occupation, the myope tends to pick those in which individual achievement—rather than team effort—is prized. You get on the honor roll in school by yourself, and the myope is a loner, anyway. He has to be to get all that reading done. The lonely intellectual pursuits such as author, journalist, architect and scholar are favored.

One researcher found that the tolerance for anxiety that myopes exhibit leads them to "sit things out" in a high-stress situation rather than to take action, and that they tend to be cautious, doubting, and compliant, and generally attempt to avoid potentially troubling situations and topics. Rather than react emotionally and fight, they'll walk away.

The typical myope, then, will do well in school, although some develop myopia in the struggle to achieve, but will only attain average grades. He will delight in his high test scores, and, because his language skill is so highly developed, enjoy proving his point in the classroom. He will of necessity spend a lot of time by himself reading and studying and concentrating on what the information *means to him.*

Taken out of that context, he will carry this introspection over into his social life, usually limited to a few friends of similar interests. They will spend a great deal of time verbalizing their recently acquired information, taking it apart, bit by bit—analyzing it—and along the way analyzing themselves. Emotions, too, can be put under this introspective microscope for examination, rather than just being experienced. Thus they are seen in a light where they are intellectually interesting, something to be examined and analyzed, rather than requiring action. Since abstractions tend to be analyses of situations, it is not at all surprising that this generation is one in which analyzing feelings through psychotherapy is seen as the way to control them.

When the myope is in trouble, he needs other people, if only to listen to him. And he needs encouragement that what he is doing is all right. It is almost as if this vestige of needing other people is an affirmation of his place in the ebb and flow of life, since he has cut himself off from the kind of empathy with others that comes through participation in sports and other social activities. You see—and he would be the first to tell you—he's not a joiner.

Of course, most myopes will not be the pure, undiluted type described here, but will exhibit some of the characteristics and not others, or have them to a greater or lesser degree. That peppy, pretty cheerleader may also be a scholastic achiever and end up nearsighted, along with the rest of us who didn't make the squad.

As for the current trend to physical fitness, it could be viewed as this era's reaction to those years of childhood when sedentary activities took up most of the day, and which led to sedentary occupations. But do myopes form a basketball team? Not likely. Jogging or skiing is the thing. You can do it anytime you want, and all by yourself. You don't need a buddy, you compete against yourself.

Interestingly enough, there is some correlation between body types and personality, which can be viewed as one more example of body and mind operating as a matched set. It appears that in the grand scheme, if you get one from column A (a certain disposition) you are probably going to get one from column B (a body type which matches). These studies were made in the late 30s and the 40s, with little follow-up since, and today many question their validity. However, the correlation appears to be borne out in R.K.'s practice: myopes tend to be tall and thin, farsighted people shorter and stockier.

It has been suggested that the myope is more sensitive to light than others, prefers a low level of visual stimulation and may unconsciously choose to tone down his acuity to enhance this. It could also be the reason that many writers and scholars prefer the quiet of the night to do their most efficient work, without the visual distractions present during the light of the day. At night you can control the visual stimulation with the flick of a switch, and the confirmed myope also is aware that to achieve results from intense, concentrated efforts, he is going to have to push past the point where his eyes send him the message they are tired.

The question is, naturally, did the disposition—put there through genetics—influence one's behavior so that myopia resulted? Or can the behavioral characteristics be seen as an outgrowth of myopia?

Child psychologists and educators have long observed that the disposition toward a certain personality type is often evident at birth. An infant can be characterized as either quiet and a "good" baby, that is, one who doesn't cause a lot of trouble, or a boisterous, rowdy type who makes a lot of noise. Although for many years the behavioral school of thought placed an inordinate emphasis on the importance of environment—how a child was reared—the pendulum is swinging back to somewhere around midpoint, where we believe it belongs.

A recent study at the University of Minnesota concludes that children are born with predispositions toward certain interests, and what parents do is of relatively little importance. The study included both teenagers reared in their natural homes, and another group raised in adoptive homes. The two groups were similar in education and income. The psychologists found a good deal of similarity between parents and children in homes where the biological connection was unbroken, but in the adoptive families the similarities were not greater than if the teenagers and parents had been chosen at random from the general population.

We feel that the difference in the adoptive relationship may be due to the child's inherited intelligence and traits being at odds with the parents'; in a natural parent-child situation, the two may be compatible and interact smoothly. Of course, the environment can and often does modify the genetic predisposition.

A child cannot aspire to become a ballet dancer unless she first sees a performance, or reads about it. Anna Pavlova saw her first performance of a ballet when she was eight and announced that day that she would become a dancer. It turned out that her lithe and supple body provided the raw materials she needed to become one of the greatest ballerinas of all time.

Our culture is such today that the skills in which near-point vision is utilized almost constantly are highly prized. Increasing technology and the trend to specialization in occupation have the effect of making us concentrate on the minutiae of life. And such meticulous fine-tuning is precisely one of the traits noticed in myopes.

Yet we cannot adapt to our changing environment in the blink of an eye, and as a result our eyes are becoming trapped in evolutionary obsolescence. Modern life demands a great deal of our eyes, and there's no reason to expect that the stress won't take its toll. The statistics tell us it already is. Remember, our eyes developed for long-distance viewing, to hunt and to farm, and not to spend hours staring at small marks on a page, be they numbers or letters. (If you, for example, have been reading right along, it's certainly time to stop and look out the window for a minute. Breathe deeply and rest your eyes.)

The counterculture revolution and its disdain for high achievement was perhaps no more than a reaction to the fact that our bodies are not really up to the visual tasks we are asking of them. The dropouts went sunning at Big Sur, skiing in Aspen, surfing in Hawaii, and whether or not one took a book along was immaterial. There would be friends and conversation and physical activity out in the sunshine, just as our ancestors' times. For a decade or so, a whole lot of people decided that the climb up the money and success and power ladder was not worth the trouble, the stress and the strain it required.

Today many of the dropouts have returned to the grind of "making it." Yet there is a difference in their perspective. They recognize the point past which it is not worth the push, and our culture today is better off because of that. The dropouts put on the brakes and taught the rest of us to slow down. It may be significant that heart attacks and strokes are on the decline among the well-educated middle class.

We are not suggesting here that the eyes are responsible for every aspect of ourselves, but they are the means through which we get 80 or 90 percent of our information about the world, and thus they are a major factor in who we are, what we do and what we will become.

Neither are we suggesting that vision therapy can change your world. We are saying that it can make a difference.

Vision therapy cannot take the shy introvert and turn him into the life of the party, but because behavior is exacerbated by a physical problem, clearing up the problem is likely to modify behavior along parallel lines.

A youngster who is not picked for the team of necessity withdraws into himself; the woman who thinks that every humorous remark is critical is not likely to join in the laughter with others. Change the vision—or return it to normal—and the person is likely to become less introverted and defensive.

Dyslexia

A few years ago an eight-year-old boy who was reading at the first-grade level rather than keeping up with his third-grade classmates came in for an examination. He would mix up *b* with *d,* see *saw* when it said *was,* read *no* for *on.* He wrote the same way. He was sensitive and lovable, but disorganized to the point where he couldn't concentrate long enough to tie a shoelace. He often wandered around and would forget what he was supposed to be doing, causing his parents a great deal of frustration. He was poor in sports, always the last one chosen when sides were drawn up for a game.

The visual examination showed that his eyes actually lost the target when an object shifted from the left side of his body to the right. He lost visual contact with it until the other eye could locate it. Consequently, the two sides of his body were not cooperating smoothly, but always as if one were fighting with the other.

He immediately perked up once he was told that something specific was the problem, and that he could do something about it. He was given a program of "games" to be done at home with his parents. The daily sessions lasted from 15 to 20 minutes, and consisted of four or five exercises aimed at getting him to coordinate the right and left sides of his body with his eyes, and asking his eyes to guide body coordination.

He did "slap-tap" procedures, which were like the clapping and tapping games children often design for themselves; he was asked to copy the alphabet on a blackboard with the right hand, but writing the letters so that they were in front of the left side of his body. He came to the office every two weeks.

Improvement was seen the second time he came. He was happier, more outgoing. By the third and fourth sessions, he was reporting—with great enthusiasm—his newly found sports ability. One time he batted a home run and won the game! Another time he was the first chosen for the team! And then suddenly it was as if the plug was pulled. After four months of therapy his reading ability shot up to his grade level, and his aptitude for other subjects put him near the top of his classes. Total visits to the doctor's office: eight. Total time elapsed: four months. Although his story seems like a miracle, it did happen. But such quick and easy "cures" do not happen all the time. Just sometimes.

We realize that the case studies presented throughout the book make vision therapy sound like a cure for everything. The stories, chosen to illustrate how vision therapy can work, are true, but not all cases are as dramatic or the results as encouraging. Vision therapy has wide-ranging effects because our eyes are responsible for so much; but it is not a panacea for all that ails us today, visual or otherwise.

By most standards, that youngster was classified as dyslexic, a condition that educators, psychologists, and neurologists find frustrating, since there appears to be no organic damage to the brain in most cases. What is frequently found is that the visual problems interfere with comprehension, but once the visual skills are refined, comprehension follows.

In practice, it is found that between 60 and 80 percent of the children who have been classified dyslexic have visual problems which are frequently combined with auditory difficulties, adding to their confusion in comprehending both written and spoken language. Language therapy, which attempts to teach the ears how to listen right just as vision therapy teaches eyes how to see right, is frequently suggested when a problem exists in both senses. People who do this work often refer to themselves as communication therapists.

Dyslexia does not usually go away of its own accord, and it can follow otherwise bright individuals throughout their lives. Well-known dyslexics who learned to cope include Nelson Rockefeller, Albert Einstein and Thomas Edison. At Harvard, dyslexics are allowed to take their examinations on a typewriter, which for some reason significantly helps their scores.

But many who fall into the loose category of dyslexia never achieve well enough to go to college at all. If the problem is severe enough they will never learn how to read.

If you can't read, you do poorly in school, which often leads to pervasive anxiety. Failure is a prime source of stress and ages us rapidly, indicating that choosing an occupation we can be good at is crucial to a long and happy life. If you can't read and write, you can always learn how to hold up a gas station or a bank, which may be one explanation for the fact that an extremely high percentage of juvenile delinquents are non-readers. The same is true of the prison population.

Roger T. Dowis, an optometrist in Boulder, Colorado may have found a way to reverse the treadmill many juvenile delinquents travel. Of the 48 youths of the Lookout Mountain School he treated with vision

therapy only 2 (or 4 percent) were returned to the school after their release, compared with 18 percent of the total school population during
the 11 months of the study.

Dr. Dowis found that 90 percent of the 444 youths he examined
in the school had learning disabilities of one sort or another involving
vision, hearing, and various sociological and psychological problems.
Most of them were almost three grade-levels below their age group. Yet
a great many of these youngsters had normal acuity, the only skill most
examinations test. What does not show up there are the difficulties in eye
tracking, focusing and teaming, which lead to the inability to concentrate and comprehend what is being looked at.

Fortunately, not all adolescents with vision problems turn to delinquency. Some just plod along year after year, unable to achieve in a
society where reading is almost as necessary as breathing. Take the case
of a 38-year-old handyman in an apartment building. He had recently
married and wanted desperately to move into a better job, but his inability to read anything beyond his name kept him back.

He had put years of effort into trying to learn how to read. When
he was a child his parents had sent him to special summer camps with
remedial reading programs. He had been in psychotherapy, but that
didn't help his problem, and the reading courses he tried again and
again failed. He could do math in his head, but couldn't make sense of it
on paper. He had to make a special arrangement with the bank so he
could write checks. He had never been able to drive a car because he
couldn't pass the driver's written test or read street signs.

When his wife read him an article on how some children were
helped with their reading difficulties by vision therapy, he made an ap-
pointment. On his first visit a simple test showed that he was intellectually grabbing for the rules about reading that had been hammered into
his head through the years. He tried to break the words down into their
individual sounds, but instead of succeeding he would simply stammer
and sweat profusely. He was not willing to give up, but his frustration was
crippling him. On a verbal intelligence test he scored in the low range of
normal. His speaking vocabulary was limited, because the means by
which the rest of us enrich ours—reading—had been denied him.

He began vision therapy, a part of which was designed to expand
his visual memory and sight vocabulary. Instead of breaking up the
words into sounds, he was encouraged to picture the word in his mind
without verbalizing. This helped him unlock the logjam which occurred
when he tried to read the phonetic way. Within six months he was reading at a third-grade level, which may not sound like much but repre-

sented a victory for the man who had lived a life of repeated failure and frustration.

At that point he was referred to a remedial reading program, the same kind which he had tried before but without success. Vision training stopped for the time. In a few months he was reading at the eighth-grade level and had a new job as an office clerk. He got his driver's license, bought a car, and he and his wife drove to Florida.

A year after his first visit he began therapy again. He wanted to go to school to become a television repairman but was still unable to follow written instructions. He could not visualize actually doing what he read. (A person who has trouble reading a road map without constantly turning it to orient himself, or someone who can't follow a recipe probably has the same difficulty with *visualization*.)

This time, visual memory skills and visualization were emphasized. An image was flashed on a screen for an instant, and he was asked to draw it. Or he was told to draw an object from different perspectives. With practice, it became easier. After training for four months he was able to enroll in the course, and eventually became a TV repairman.

Although he had been classified a dyslexic most of his life, and was thought to have minimal brain damage, the difficulty was simply that he never properly learned how to use his visual abilities. He could not look at symbols and transform them into meaning. They remained unintelligible forms on a page until he was taught how to see.

Problems which show up most frequently in people who have difficulty reading are those of tracking (following a line across a page smoothly), focusing (tuning in on one particular form or word), and teaming (working the eyes together smoothly). The signal to the brain has so much static zapping around that a person cannot comprehend what is being reported—and what's going on.

At the same time, it is likely that the person's ability to interpret what is being seen by perceiving similarities and differences never developed fast enough to keep up with the needs for school tasks, eventually causing so much anxiety that the child simply gave up. This is in contrast to the myopic person, who will often push past the pain of tired eyes, and maybe even headaches, and keep on going.

Learning to read is similar to learning to see. First, an infant develops a visual vocabulary for objects—mama's face, the crib, the spoon. Second, talking brings in another aspect: *things have names.* So do colors. In time our vocabulary teaches us that horses are not blue, that a black horse is similar to a brown horse is similar to a white horse. The child understands the large concept into which many small ones fit.

How this works can perhaps best be explained by how it can go wrong, as in this true story: A mother and her four-year-old son were in a concentration camp in Germany during World War II. One day as they stood by the barbed wire fence, there was a horse grazing on the other side. There were *no fences around him.* "That's freedom," the mother said, including in her gaze the wide expanse of sky, the field, the horse.

Mother and son survived the war. After they were freed, they came upon a horse in his stall.

The boy pointed and said, "That's freedom."

By the time a child is ready to take the step to read, his visual vocabulary needs to be in good working order so he can take the jump to the next level of the learning process: abstraction. Making the lines and shapes which spell *horse* means that big animal which runs fast, makes noise, likes to eat carrots and looks like the wooden character on the merry-go-round that goes up and down.

In time, the words fit into sequences with other words. The reader learns how to manipulate them so that *May I play with the ball?* has a different meaning from *I may play with the ball,* even though the words are the same. The order is different. A visual interference may prevent this difference in meaning from being understood; an auditory imbalance may do likewise.

Even people who are extremely bright can have these problems, as did a ninth-grader who scored over 140 on I.Q. tests—as long as the test was oral or untimed. He was several years behind his classmates in reading, with grades well below average. A severe facial tic made it difficult to look at him and carry on a conversation without being distracted. Weekly visits to a psychiatrist brought no relief except a prescription for a tranquilizer. Several neurological workups could not isolate the problem. Everyone continued to tell him he was extremely bright, so why couldn't he read fast enough to pass a written test?

The pressure to succeed—when he was told over and over again that he had the ability—led to other emotional problems. He thought people were "out to get him." They kept telling him he was bright when it was obvious to him that he couldn't be. He was distrustful of others and unhappy with himself. In school, when he was annoyed, he would simply get up and walk out. He couldn't take it any longer.

A school psychologist eventually suggested that he have a visual examination by a behavioral optometrist. What showed up were problems in eye tracking and teaming. He couldn't follow a line across a page smoothly, and his eyes were operating independently. Extensive vision therapy was begun. He came to the office between two and three times a week. No special reading training was suggested.

Within a year he was reading at three or more years above his class level. His grades jumped from low scores to the top of the class. He was pleased with himself academically, and no longer found it necessary to walk out of class when he was agitated—he didn't get that upset anymore.

While the tic was alleviated somewhat, he had it still. Other aspects of his ingrained and antisocial behavior remained. It was hard for him to learn to trust anybody, and in turn, it was hard to like him. Although he had smoothed out the academic wrinkles in his life, the emotional scars from years of frustration and anxiety remained. Had he been seen earlier, perhaps he would have recovered more completely.

It is easier to prevent than to cure.

Farsightedness or Hyperopia

When we consider how the eye evolved in man, it is not surprising that approximately 75 percent of the world's population has a small amount of farsightedness, or hyperopia. Distance vision was most valuable to man as he hunted or looked for plants he could eat. When he began tending his own crops, he still did not spend long stretches of time concentrated on near-point focus. Since the greater proportion of the world's population is farsighted, it is our calculations which must be off, for the majority should be the norm, and not have a label pinned on them which sounds as if something is wrong.

In healthy vision a person can easily adjust his focus from a point in the distance to a point up close. The focus moves from behind the retina to directly on it; there is no difficulty in shifting it, such as the myopic person experiences.

If a person has what is called *absolute hyperopia,* the focus stays

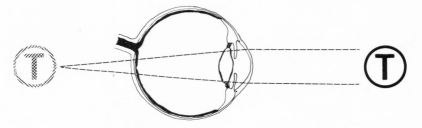

Hyperopia occurs when an image focuses behind the retina.

behind the retina. While the evidence indicates that myopia is the result of the environment, the causes of absolute hyperopia are much less clear. It may be linked to other congenital deformities, such as mental retardation, where hyperopia is prevalent. Other causes appear to be related to high fever and serious illness during the early years.

The behavior associated with farsighted individuals is not the exact opposite of that connected with myopes, possibly because myopia is an aberration, and a certain degree of farsightedness is not. Research has shown that moderately farsighted individuals tend to be more concerned about tomorrow than the here and the now, or the past. They are generally extroverted, need to know what others are thinking, and listen to their suggestions. Due to their gregarious natures they will often be the center of activity—but on the playing field rather than the chess club. They like overall organization and structure but tend to gloss over details.

For instance, in planning a trip, say a romantic second honeymoon to Bermuda, the hyperope will call the travel agent, make the reservations, pick up the tickets, arrange for the rental car, pack ahead of time, and get to the airport two hours early. Plenty of time to check in and have a leisurely drink. Since everything is already taken care of, the hyperope will sit back and relax. He will be so relaxed he will not notice that all those people walking by are probably going to . . . Bermuda. And he will miss the plane by five minutes! Fortunately for R.K., the farsighted romantic lead in this scenario, another airline had a plane leaving an hour later. They made it.

The hyperopes' need for change leads them to find studying and reading boring after a while, and thus they are less dedicated students. However, there is no evidence that they are not as intelligent as myopes; they just go at it differently.

They enjoy team sports, and later on this rah-rah group activity is transferred to occupational choices, frequently leading them to professions where teamwork is prized: business. Remember too, that since the fine points of academia fail to fascinate, the variety of stimuli in business—calling on clients, board meetings, dictating letters, preparing reports—offers a pleasant choice. A nearsighted secretary can take care of the details.

Because of the long hours of solitude demanded by those pursuits where individual achievement is critical, the farsighted person tends to end up in professions which do not have high status in our culture, where professor, judge and doctor are synonymous with status.

Since they tend to lose details in the overall structure, hyperopes do not differentiate among people, places, and words as much as do myopes. Therefore they do not score as high on academic memory tests but have good recall for personal events and feelings. Typically, one will remember what happened between Alfred and Mary Kate last summer when they stayed on the *Queen Mary,* probably because he empathizes with feelings to a marked degree, especially when compared with his nearsighted counterpart.

With their focus on similarities rather than differences, farsighted individuals may consider specific requests tedious and unnecessary, and be lax in complying with them. Not surprisingly, hyperopes are more difficult to collect data on than myopes.

In a 1968 study at the Virginia Military Institute designed to show the relationship between behavior and vision, roughly two-thirds of the subjects who had to be dropped due to lack of data were non-myopes. Among the findings (from which some of the above observations came) was that more than twice as many myopes became officers, as compared to non-myopes.

Because ours is a culture which depends on the details and differences inherent in today's technology, the individual who is bored by them is at a disadvantage. There is an unusually high percentage of farsighted individuals among the dyslexic population, and this is particularly true with groups of juvenile delinquents or the inmates of prisons. It could be that in our society, where intellect and the almighty buck are prized, those who can't compete normally become angry with the situation and, unable to change it, strike out against society.

The sad fact is that if they had been discovered early and given help before the frustration of repeated failure set in, they might have been able to develop those skills which are more compatible with a smooth and easy life in the twentieth century.

Yet children with difficulty sustaining near-point focusing may not be discovered, since they are able to do it just long enough for a visual examination, and other aberrations go unnoticed. Unfortunately, the consensus continues to be that if a child can read enough letters on a chart, there's no problem with vision.

Presbyopia
A type of farsightedness which afflicts all of us to a greater or lesser degree as we get older is called *presbyopia.* What happens is that the involuntary nervous system, which has been in charge of focusing

without your being aware that anything is going on, and the voluntary nervous system, which directs the eye when you want to look at something, age at varying rates. In their younger days, they work well together, each allowing the other a bit of freedom. It's a happy marriage. If they got out of step a bit, no one—including the owner—was the wiser. Sight was easy.

As we age, however, there is a wider and wider gap in their two-step. The voluntary system declines slowly, but the involuntary system starts going downhill somewhere in our teens or earlier. This gap usually goes unnoticed for a quarter of a century, but somewhere in the mid-thirties or thereabouts it begins to cause trouble, which may *not* be noticed at first as a difficulty in seeing. Reading speed and efficiency slow down; a typist makes more errors, and mistakes creep in when adding up a list of numbers. We're aging.

More likely than not, a person will find one day when he *voluntarily* aims his eyes at an object—say, a printed page—that the image is fuzzy. The worn down, *involuntary* system isn't keeping up, and the image that goes to the brain doesn't have sharp definition. It is seen as a blur. The brain sends out a signal to *try harder,* the stress juices get flowing, resulting in greater wear and tear on the system. Short of giving up crocheting, reading and bridge, is there anything which can be done besides glasses?

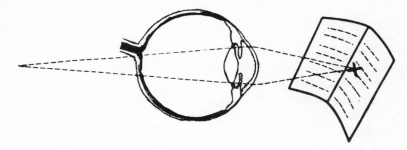

Presbyopia takes place when the image for close objects is behind the retina.

One woman was determined to find out. A television personality in her late fifties, she didn't want to begin wearing glasses or contact lenses. Yet it was obvious to her that her vision was failing. After reading an article about vision training, she came for an examination and outlined her goal: reading without glasses. Three months later she was having no trouble doing so.

Her acuity jumped from 20/200 to 20/30—in good light.

Her success story is highly unusual. Such therapy is successful to this degree only about five percent of the time.

In poor light, however, she experiences difficulty. In fact, lowering the lighting is one of the tools she uses to train her vision. In lower illumination the pupil enlarges to let more light in. However, this has the effect of also enlarging the blurred image. She thereby developed the ability to interpret blurred words and images better. Turn up the light and the pupil constricts, the image does the same and appears sharper than before.

You can demonstrate the effects of constricting the pupil by taking a piece of cardboard and putting a pinhole in the center. Take off your glasses, look through the pinhole and you will see almost as clearly as with your glasses.

To maintain her improved vision—and to keep away from using her dreaded glasses—she needs remedial therapy every 18 months or so, for eight to 10 weeks. Therapy seems to arrest the deteriorating condition for a while, but then the old wheel of time keeps revolving. A key factor in her success appears to be her high motivation, which is crucial to all aspects of vision therapy, but especially when treating presbyopia. It's just like going on a diet. Losing weight and improving visual skills are not done *to* you—you have to make the decision that they are worth the time and trouble and then proceed.

Other older individuals may see clearly when reading, but still be uncomfortable. Some who have been avid readers lose interest in life itself when they are unable to easily keep up the reading they enjoy. One man, who had looked forward to retirement so that he would have the time to read all the books in his library, found to his dismay that he couldn't. It was too hard. He was severely depressed: what was he going to do with the rest of his life? Vision therapy gave him a new outlook and sent him back to the stacks.

Astigmatism

Close to 80 percent of the population have eyes which are not perfect spheres. But it is only when the structure is so disproportionately out of shape that it causes focusing difficulty. Light rays coming in become bent at different angles, depending on the distortion of the particular places they strike the eye. These different angles scatter the focus and the brain can't decode the garbled message. Since the information does not come to a single focus, reaching a decision about what is seen is less than simple. Straight lines may appear crooked, people can look

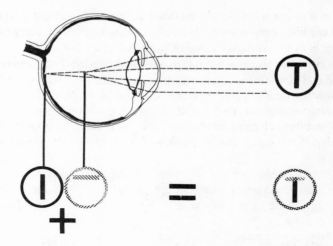

Simple myopic astigmatism occurs when one image focus is on
the retina and a second image is in front of the retina.

longer or squatter than they are, vertical lines may be clear while
horizontal ones shimmer.

As with so many other misconceptions about our eyes, it has generally been believed that astigmatism was inherited and fixed, but
studies at the Gesell Institute show that it often varies during the early
years. Astigmatism that is measured at age one disappears entirely, only

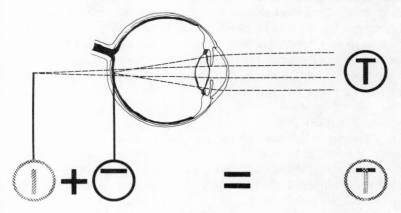

Simple hyperopic astigmatism takes place when one image
focus is on the retina and a second image is behind the retina.

to return at another date. And sometimes youngsters who are astigmatic to a degree which would cause difficulty can be helped to a degree, although this is one of the least effective types of therapy.

Understanding how astigmatism develops can be instrumental in preventing it. If posture is tilted, or the face misshapen, the eyes will attempt to allow for the distortion and try their best to maintain a correct balance, straining some muscles, relaxing others.

How a physical imbalance can lead to optical distortions is understandable if we imagine that the body is composed of triangles bal-

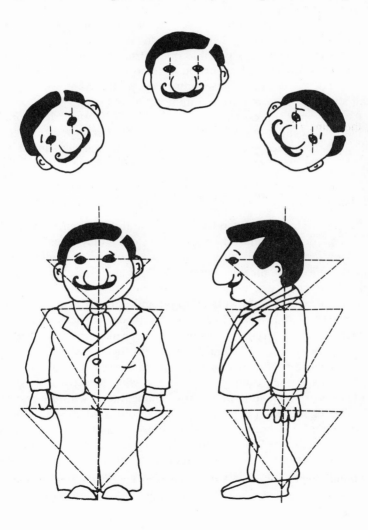

ancing on top of one another. If one of the triangles is not balanced, the others won't be, either.

Now if one part of the body is warped, the head is going to try to compensate to keep everything at an even keel. So now the head is tilted, and the eyes do their best to make up for that. *Hey you, straighten out! Don't you know it's hard to see this way? You don't notice it, you say—huh! You ought to try the view from here! Okay, I'll go along with your crazy posture—I'll stretch myself out of shape to accommodate it. But then I won't work as well when you sit up straight or walk around. You can't have everything, you know.*

A fair number of children have cranial and facial distortions when they are born, but usually these level out in a few years so that the adult appears normal. It is possible that during the time when vision is developing, these physical distortions—which may be slight enough that they will not be noticed—cause unnecessary stress and strain on the eyeball and push the eye into becoming astigmatic.

At this stage of development, the brain's feature detectors, the little bodies of cells that get activated when a certain type of image (up, down, around, or across) comes in, are getting warmed up. If something limits the scope of possibilities to be tested, some of the detectors will wither or change. If the horizontal images aren't coming in clearly, the feature detector for horizontals doesn't learn how to work properly, and so on through the spectrum.

For example, Zulus, who live in a circular environment with round huts, round doors, round shapes, round tools—they even plow their fields in curves—have difficulty making sense of sharp angles and perpendicular lines. When called upon to look at angles, Zulus become disoriented and confused, and because of this they cannot understand drawings and photographs with sharp up-and-down edges.

Research with animals backs up this theory. Kittens raised in environments where everything was on a vertical plane became insensitive to other types of lines and would bump into them; they could not perceive what those other lines meant. If a child is born with a facial distortion—perhaps the result of a delivery with forceps—it is possible that the eyes are bent somewhat out of shape, along with the rest of the head. The light rays, entering the eye at distorted points, would be bent irregularly and not come to a single focus, and would therefore be perceived indistinctly. The feature detectors responsible for those types of lines would atrophy, or perhaps tune in to other contours and planes. The individual would be left with an insensitivity to a certain type of line, unless the problem corrects itself, or does so with help. Before the age of four drastic changes are possible, as the following case demonstrates.

Johnny was 18 months old when his mother first brought him for an examination. He held the right side of his body stiffly. His right foot turned in. When he walked he held his right hand awkwardly at his side, while the left hand swung freely. His eyes did not appear to be "right." His mother had been in vision therapy herself, and thought the problem might be related to his vision. Although his fingers were dexterous, his whole body movement was clumsy. The examination indicated that he was astigmatic in the right eye.

Exercises were designed for him to do daily at home with his mother. These alternately used each side of his body, with his eyes steering the movements. He climbed up and down stairs and took each step with the opposite foot. He walked through a series of hoops on the floor. He crawled through a tunnel.

A few months later the astigmatism was reduced to the norm, and his body movements were coordinated. The foot no longer turned in as much.

Some cases of astigmatism are helped by having the person wear weaker and weaker glasses. The eye attempts to make up the missing boost it had been getting from the glasses. Since each prescription is only slightly weaker, the eyes are not strained unduly, so they try to meet the task. Every few months the lenses are changed.

This is what was prescribed for a five-year-old whose astigmatism was relatively mild. No body work was suggested, but his eyeglasses were changed for ones which did not compensate as much as his old ones. His eyes took up the gap. Weaker glasses were prescribed again. Once more, the eyes rose to the occasion. Over a period of six months, the glasses were changed four times. No fifth pair was needed.

We have used an unusual and dramatic example to illustrate that vision therapy, in some cases, can reduce or eliminate optical distortions, but we wish to emphasize that this is rare and extremely difficult, once the distortion has become fixed.

As with all vision therapy, it works because the person is motivated. It is not something which can be done to you, like plugging in an electric gadget to lose weight. Of course, what is possible varies from person to person. Age and lifelong habits of perceiving in a certain way, reacting a certain way, sometimes can prevent real change. However, as some case studies indicate, that is not necessarily true. Motivation is always a factor, as is the severity of the problem. And it is always easier to prevent problems than to eliminate them.

Nonetheless, even correcting astigmatism, which is the result of measurable structural change, has been accomplished in adults on a few occasions. A reading specialist in her mid-forties had worn glasses for astigmatism and myopia most of her life. She decided to find out what could be done for herself in vision therapy, since so many of her students with perceptual problems had benefited from it. Besides, she was tired of wearing glasses—and now they were getting thicker and less attractive. Even the most stylish frames couldn't make up for that.

Her acuity was 20/200. Her astigmatism measured five units in each eye (.75 is normal). After 10 months of therapy the teacher who had always worn glasses was able to go without them most of the time. Her acuity tested at anywhere from 20/30 to 20/60. And her astigmatism was reduced by a unit.

It is true that the shape of her eyeball was not highly malleable due to age, but astigmatism sometimes responds to therapy. The same is true in all aspects of vision therapy: the earlier the better. If a maladaptation—such as an eye which wanders only sometimes—is caught early enough, it is usually simple to right it. An eye which turns in once in a while does not have to become a crossed eye. It's as if a child got on the wrong train at the station; instead of going to Phoenix, he's headed for Pittsburgh. Better retrieve him before he gets too far. And with early correction, the psychological effects don't have a chance to get entrenched.

Extensive studies with schoolchildren in Texas some 40 years ago clearly demonstrated how lighting can affect posture, which in turn can affect vision. In all, some 160,000 children in 4,000 classrooms were involved. What was discovered was that a child at work unconsciously shifts his head and body to reduce glare or shadows. This can eventually distort the skeletal structure, leading to visual difficulties and other physical complaints.

At the Becker School in Austin close to 400 children were given complete physical and visual examinations as well as standardized achievement tests in November of 1942. More than 50 percent of them had visual difficulties which appeared to be related to their achievement scores.

Then several changes in their school environment were made. The seating arrangements were changed from the straight rows to groups, so that all the desks in the classroom received the same amount of light. The lighting was modified, the walls repainted a restful, glare-free color.

In May the children were examined again. Less than 20 percent still had visual problems, *a drop of 30 percent*. The other medical findings showed a sharp decline in chronic fatigue and ear, nose and throat infections. While the two might not seem to be related, such respiratory infections may be the result of a lack of adequate Vitamin A, which is consumed by the eyes in inordinate amounts when lighting is low or glare is present.

Scholastically, the students grew faster than their peers at other schools where no lighting or seating changes were made; at the end of six months, the children in the Becker School were more than three months ahead.

Darell Boyd Harmon, a design consultant more interested in the effect of interiors than their appearance, did a study for the Texas State Health Department. As part of the work, he devised a simple test to determine whether optical distortions were present. Take a standard piece of unlined paper and as quickly as you can—without glasses—draw three rows of squares approximately the same size as your handwriting across the page. The result will reveal if your perception of space is distorted. If you are astigmatic, the boxes will run across the page at a tilt, or will be asymmetrical. Yet, if a person without astigmatism looks at the boxes through special glasses designed for the degree of astigmatism, they will look nearly square and in a straight line. In a similar way, the elongated figures of El Greco and Hans Holbein appear normal when viewed through glasses for astigmatism.

Besides sight, another job of the eyes is to help keep the world in its proper perspective when you walk around. Although balance is primarily a function of the inner ear, vision's job is to keep the horizon level. When it is not, the whole eye/ear/body coordinating system goes out of whack, just as it does on a rocking boat. When this motion-caused dizziness and disorientation start the stress juices flowing, simply press down on the balls of your feet to tell your body where it is. Often that will allay the distress.

Until NASA figured out how to compensate for the difficulty, the astronauts on the early flights suffered similar disorientation. Gravity wasn't around to tell the body where it was—or where the horizon was.

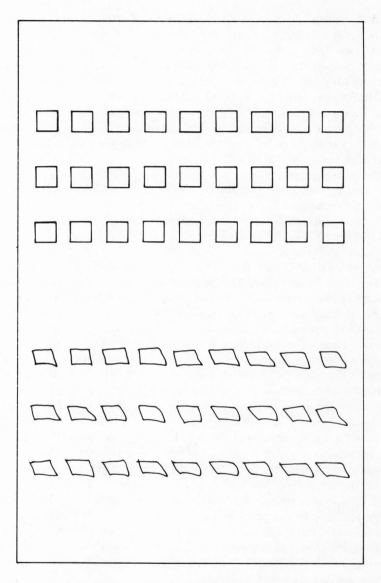

Since the astigmatic eyeball is irregular, a person with horizontal astigmatism will have difficulty perceiving horizontal lines. A tall building will look fine, but letters running across a page might get jumbled, since the cross in a *t* will be unclear, while the vertical *l* will be easily seen. In sports, fly balls will be a snap to catch while the low ground balls zip right past.

Although the literature on how astigmatism relates to behavior is sketchy, in practice it has been observed that astigmatic people have a difficult time coming to a decision and then taking action. It is not simply that they see two points of view—they may know what they want to do, but focusing on it long enough to actually get moving seems difficult.

Do you have a friend who makes a lot of decisions based on the toss of a coin? Ask him why he wears his glasses. But remember the Chinese believe that it matters not how you acquire self-knowledge, as long as you do; and anyway, once the coin is in the air, you will usually be aware how you want it to land.

Crossed Eyes or Strabismus

Through the crack of a door one has limited outlook; one looks outward from within. Contemplation is subjectively limited. One tends to relate everything to oneself and cannot put oneself in another's place and understand his motives.

"I have an eye that crosses when I'm tired or nuts."—*The New York Times,* April 15, 1977. The speaker is someone whose stunning face grins out of the pages of many magazines these days. Model and actress Lauren Hutton, the woman who made having a space between her two front teeth practically fashionable, is not likely to do that for crossed eyes.

Although many other eye defects are more serious in their effect on perception, few are as troubling as strabismus, since crossed eyes are distracting to the viewer. It is a deformity parents can see, and they have the vague idea that it is correctible.

Unfortunately, far too many children end up on the operating table for surgery that in a high percentage of cases is unsuccessful. Oh, the eye may straighten for a while, and child and parents are pleased. But over a period of months the same inward or outward turning of the eye reappears. Surgery is often repeated, sometimes even a third time before the eye stays straight. It has simply given up.

Few operations are as unnecessary or have such disastrous results —even when the eye appears straight. The child sees that his eye appears straight. He's happy, his parents are pleased. All that money wasn't wasted. But now, why does he have double vision? Is that the way everybody sees? Why is he always bumping into things? What's wrong? The child is more confused than ever, afraid that indeed something is different about him. And they said the operation would make it right.

In addition, there is the shock of surgery, which is always an assault on the body, and there is the possibility of accidental death due to other complications. One study at a New York City hospital puts the number of deaths at approximately 7 in 3,500 eye operations of all types.

And the rate of success—two eyes which function together—is only *20 percent,* as reported in the surgical literature. Although the eye may appear straight, in the vast majority of cases it does not function as it should. The child may develop *amblyopia,* which is a shutting down of the perceptual center where the visual information is received from the eye. The person is now, for all intents and purposes, blind in one eye when he tries to see with both, or the problem may be deflected to another muscle.

Yet through vision therapy—and this data is from sources all over the world—the rate of success is *75 percent.*

So why do surgeons continue to cut? Because they are trained to. And because the old idea of why eyes cross is still rampant today, even though the scientific information belies this. Change, as we have noted, comes slowly.

The traditional idea is that of the six muscles moving the eyeball, some are stronger than others and pull the eye one way, overcoming the force of the muscles going the other way. Yet we know that each muscle has at least 50 to 100 times the strength it needs to move an eyeball around. Surgery attempts to reattach the muscle tendon at some other place on the eyeball, thereby straightening it. Unsuccessful surgery may make it impossible for the eye/brain mechanism ever to right itself. Each cutting leaves more and more scar tissue.

One little girl came in after she had had two operations. True, her right eye didn't turn in anymore—now it turned up and out. The eye began turning in when she was a year old. The family doctor said she would outgrow it. But it still turned in at age four, and this time the family went ahead with surgery. It worked—for a while. At seven, the eye turned in again. A second operation was seemingly successful. For an entire week, the eye appeared straight.

And then it went up and out, leaving a patch of white where one shouldn't be. Surgery was suggested again, but this time the parents refused, and the ophthalmologist suggested they take the child to a vision therapist.

On examination it was found that she had limited movement and severely weakened vision in that eye—conditions which frequently accompany an eye that turns in or out. Her focus did not fall on the *macula* of the eye, that concentrated patch of cones which is responsible for our clearest central vision. It was off to the side a few degrees, and anything other than dead center dims vision. It's like setting the dial of a radio not quite on the frequency.

A method of treatment being done in Europe was tried. *Pleoptics* involves light stimulation with a special instrument. The cones of the macula are darkened, while the others are flashed so much light they are temporarily out of commission. Then the patch of darkness is lifted. If the eye is to see, it must do so with the macula. Eventually it does. The eye sees as if it were looking through the hole of a donut. The girl came to the office every morning for a half hour; the procedure was done four or five times. Within a month the macula was being used, but the eye now had to learn how to see, a process it had stopped long ago.

The child had to learn how to merge what she could feel with what she saw. She had stopped melding sight and touch at age one. When she walked she often bumped into things; she had difficulty recognizing shapes which she knew through touch and had a hard time copying letters and figures.

A program of exercises was started: tracing lines, circling all the *C*s (or any other letter) in a newspaper column, putting dots in the center of letters, reading smaller and smaller letters. In a little over a year after her first visit she was able to fuse the sight from both eyes with the aid of special glasses. Her acuity improved markedly. But her eye never went completely straight. It had lost its flexibility and continued to turn up at times because of the scar tissue.

With surgery, nothing happens in the eye/brain where the problem has been all along. Strabismus—whether the eye turns in or out—is merely another way the eyes have of adapting to stress: high fevers, which disrupt the nervous system; an injury to one eye, preventing it from completing its learning process during the first six years; cataracts in one eye; swollen lids that cover the eye for weeks or months, or something as seemingly innocent as having a crib kept against one wall. If the child is sedentary and does not move around, the eye next to the wall will not be used often enough to look out across the room.

Consequently that eye gets bored and turns in: *Don't need to use this eye—nothing interesting to see.* . . .

Many patients report that they developed the problem when they were between two and three years old. The "terrible twos" are indeed difficult for most children. They are often tense, get upset easily, lose the good coordination that they had six months earlier. One moment they are over-focusing on one thing, the next moment they are onto several things all at once. Interrupt them and they will go into a tirade. And they don't like to take chances.

In practice, it is found that those children whose eyes cross at this early age are often bright, articulate, intense and addicted to a ritualistic way of doing things. Many adult patients will discuss the emotional problems they lived with at that age: their parents' divorce, death or serious illness. One man's eyes crossed during the year his mother had to place him in a foster home. He had transfered a psychological trauma to his eye.

Turning an eye in severely limits perception. A youngster may not want to deal with the world after a parent dies or leaves. He turns the eye in and tunes out. School may be too much, too soon. He gives up and turns out. *Hey—there's more to handle than I can. Don't like what I see, anyway. But I've got a way. If I do this and turn in toward my nose, I can't see as much. Think I'll do that. Oh, I know it looks funny—so what? Appearances aren't everything.*

But they do make a difference, as this young woman discovered:

The patient, who was in her late twenties, was a recognized painter. She taught at a major university. One eye tended to turn in, but not all the time; when it did, she hated the way she looked. Because she didn't want others to see her funny eye, and because she was generally depressed, she would closet herself in her room on weekends, sometimes not even going out for the newspaper. Her appearance was slovenly, the makeup nil. Her paintings were full of dark demons. She herself was tense and agitated; she took Valium to help her get through the day.

Her psychotherapist eventually suggested that she have her eyes examined by a behavioral optometrist and she started therapy. The changes which occurred within a year were remarkable. The bleak and desolate figures disappeared from her paintings, along with the muddy black and blues. Now the figures were free and floating, the colors were brighter—sunny hues could even be discovered in them.

Although she remains a reserved person, she is more outgoing and relaxed. She knows what she wants and is willing to put up a fight for it, rather than retreat into herself as she had done before when someone looked at her the wrong way. Last summer she signed up for a tour of southern France with a group of strangers. Even she recognizes she would never have done that before. She hasn't refilled her prescription for Valium: "I feel I don't want to need that anymore." And she bought some new clothes and started wearing makeup. You could call that superficial, or you could call it taking care of yourself—and caring about others and how they react to you.

Turning the eye out is much less common, but it also suppresses vision, since with all the action going on at the edges of peripheral vision, one misses what's going on in front of his nose. It is not unusual for someone with an outward-turning eye to complain that his scope of vision has narrowed once his eyes are straight. The choice to turn out is a choice to turn away from something troubling—maybe the details of learning to read and write. This often occurs at age six or seven, when the youngster begins school.

This type of person is usually not as verbal as the one who turns an eye in, yet will be highly creative and intuitive—unless those attributes were discouraged during the early years. Such a person has difficulty focusing on one thing or completing whatever he starts—something else always distracts him.

Crossed eyes can be used as attention getters. The young man described earlier, whose severely crossed eyes had kept him at home and out of the mainstream, said that his eyes first began turning in when he was six and a younger brother was born with severe physical deformities. The brother occupied his parents' attention almost entirely. Since the older boy was normal, he could fend for himself—unless he developed a problem.

He developed crossed eyes, and he was started on a program of eye exercises called *orthopics* to help strengthen the muscles. During the weekly visits to the therapist he had his mother's undivided attention. As soon as the eyes would straighten a bit and the exercises were stopped, they would begin to cross again. He needed more attention.

Many years later, when he was in psychotherapy—combined with vision therapy—he joyfully exclaimed that he could see more this time when his eyes began to straighten. But then he became a problem to the psychotherapist. The patient became petulant and demanding. Phone calls came at all times of the day or night; he wanted more attention. Since he no longer had a physical deformity, he created a psychological problem to get special attention. He was trying to make sure that he got what the eye had accomplished without words. Once he admitted this, progress in both vision therapy and psychotherapy began rolling along.

Amblyopia and Suppressed Vision

When an eye turns in, both eyes look at different objects, but the brain wants to deal with only one subject at a time—apples or oranges, but not app/ges—and so may start rejecting the *ges,* to concentrate on apples. In order to avoid the confusion, the brain ignores the inconsistent data.

The suppressed eye can perform by itself when necessary, so that this condition is not discovered when one covers the other eye. The person is not aware that he is not seeing with both eyes. In time, the dormant eye may weaken and have reduced vision, uncorrectable with glasses. This is called *amblyopia.*

A person with suppressed vision in one eye could be thought of as one dimensional. Trying to imagine what it would be like to walk in another man's shoes, or seeing another's point of view, is often difficult, if not downright impossible. When suppression continues long enough and amblyopia results, a person is left with an unbalanced way of seeing. H. G. Wells wrote in his autobiography that he believed his uneven vision, good in one eye, poor in the other, prevented him from becoming a better writer.

The story of one successful New York model illustrates how a narrowed perspective limits personality and behavior. Jamie was in her late twenties when she first came to have her eyes examined. She knew she was slightly farsighted, but she didn't have to wear glasses. She heard about vision therapy, and she just had the feeling that there might be something there for her. If you were to look her in the eyes, you wouldn't notice that one turned in slightly. She didn't know it herself, but it showed up on examination.

It was also discovered that she often blocked her vision from that eye without being aware of it. She was so used to it, and the limited perspective that it gave her, that she assumed the world looked that way to everyone. It wasn't because her eye couldn't function, for it would do fine when asked to perform by itself. It simply gave up when the other eye was on, and that was most of the time. The brain just turned off the switch for processing data from that eye.

When told what her problem was, she broke into tears. The aberration of her eye was a symbol telling her that something else inside was very wrong indeed. When she had quieted down she said that maybe that was the reason some of her photographs would be good, and then, for no apparent reason, the next one would somehow miss. Jamie brought out her book of pictures, and it was easy for R.K.'s trained eye to pick out the pictures she didn't like. He caught the slight turn of the eye.

She started therapy, and her face began to look different, as if something had been filled in. "I'm not stupid either," she rejoiced one day. She had just discovered that she could handle her checkbook. While she had been a success in front of the camera, she had never been able to handle the business of modeling. And although there was always a list of books she wanted to read, she never actually began them. Now she did. She was delighted to know that she didn't have to think of herself as "beautiful but dumb."

Something else happens when a person has amblyopia or suppressed vision. Although most of the nerve connections to and from the eyes go straight to the command center of the brain, approximately 20 percent have another job to do. They inform the body-balancing center that stabilizes us as we walk around. They make our world right side up and coordinate one side of the body with the other. Working well, they make you graceful; when they don't, it's likely you'll be clumsy—always bumping into things, knocking over glasses. The person can't quite understand why he is such a klutz.

Another mechanism that helps you see where things are in space is also hindered. To view the world in three dimensions (depth, height, and width) both eyes must work as a unit. The information coming from each one is flat; only when they are melded in the brain do we see in 3-D. If not, there are going to be a lot of unintentional bumps and grinds in your life. And you won't even know what's wrong or what you are missing.

Several months after starting vision therapy, L.D. spent a weekend in the Berkshires. On the last afternoon, a sunny fall day, she lazed away an hour or so lying on the grass under a tree and looked at the distant hills.

Everything seemed to be separated by perceptible layers of space. The tree was right by my side, and far away—really far, not just what I intellectually knew to be true—were the mountains. And way past that, high in the sky, that's where the clouds were. I lay there silently reveling in a brand new experience, looking from the tree to the mountain tops to the clouds.

A friend joined me, and I tried to explain, but he didn't

know what I was talking about, just as I wouldn't have earlier. I would have known then that the mountains were several miles away, and I thought I saw them that way, but I'd never felt the difference.

I thought: I have been missing this all of my life. What else? Vision therapy gave me many things that are perhaps more crucial to my outlook and personality, but I always remember that day as one of its most beautiful and sensual gifts.

I told the doctor and he just smiled; he'd heard the same story many times before. It happened to him once, too—at the ballet.

3
Visualizations

If a revolution is not founded on such inner truth, the re-
sults are bad, and it has no success. For in the end men will sup-
port only those undertakings which they feel instinctively to be
just.

Because we are human, each of us has the ability to create rich
and vivid imagery which we can run through our minds like scenes from
a summer night. Because we are human, each of us has what can be
called the inner eye, an ability to imagine, to visualize with the lights
out, the eyelids of night down. We can at will conjure up an image of
mother, or the first person we kissed in the movies when we were 13,
or the face of our child when she was born. This ability to visualize
people, places and events has been used since the stirring of human
consciousness to heal, to comfort, to communicate and to entertain.
In fact, the ability to imagine danger has allowed man—the naked
ape—to dominate all other species. Some of us have the ability to read
novels and create the scenes in our minds like reels of a film. And has
anyone ever found his daydreams boring?

Although the ability to visualize images in the mind appears to be
inherent in man, our technological culture with its emphasis on words
that primarily communicate thoughts instead of pictures denigrates this
very human trait to the point where some of us aren't even aware of it.
We have repressed a part of what it means to be human. We have let
logic dominate intuition; we are afraid to trust our feelings.

But we have not quite lost the ability to visualize. Only a small
percentage of the population say they do not daydream in images.
However, most people today do not take their daydreams seriously, or
work at them, or use them to make themselves feel happy and healthy.
Perhaps we repress this ability because giving in to it seems like a

75

regression to a past when there were countless phenomena man could not comprehend logically, and so he accepted and explained these in the same way he lived with the images in his head, which he knew existed, but could not explain. But in letting rationality rule we have cut down our ability for creativity that comes not in words but in pictures.

The inner eyes exists all by itself; it arrives when we are born. Children lead lives rich in imagery with their make-believe play and friends. It is thought that this is how they start learning—before abstract thought takes over and the not-so-subtle emphasis in our culture reduces the ability to play with mental pictures and watch movies in their head.

The imagery in children's play may also be a means to develop empathy with others. The child tries out how it might feel to be mom or dad or an imaginary friend. By downplaying this ability to try out different roles, perhaps we reduce the ability to empathize with others.

Some of us visualize in seemingly unlimited quality and quantity, while in others it will be minimal. Many extremely creative people are high in visualization, and may in fact have trouble communicating their concepts to others since none of the words seem right.

Einstein is a case in point. He did not learn to speak until he was three, and his speech was labored until the age of seven. He did so poorly in grammar school he was thought to be retarded. Today he would be classified dyslexic. When he transferred to another school where his non-verbal abilities were coddled, the young genius flourished. Later he would write that his concepts always came to him in images without words:

> *Words or language, as they are written or spoken, do not seem to play any role in my mechanism of thought. . . . For me it is not dubious that our thinking goes on for the most part without use of words.*

Non-verbal imagery occurs in the right hemisphere of the brain, the side which is creative, intuitive, emotional, artistic; the skills that are prized today for the most part are in the domain of the left hemisphere: logic, science, language.

How closely the eye is connected with the whole person is evident in the fact that the direction your eyes drift when you are looking for the solution to a problem is related to what kind of person you are.

When confronted with a problem or listening to information that is not easy to comprehend, we look up and away while searching our minds for the solution. People whose eyes move to the left are observed to be basically governed by their right hemisphere, and those whose eyes drift to the right are left-brained.

The eye/brain mechanism is designed so that objects in the field of vision to the left of the body's midline are dealt with by the right hemisphere. The reverse is true as well. By letting one's eyes drift to the left or the right, it is as if we are searching for the answer in the opposite hemisphere of the brain, the side with which we feel the most comfortable. It's not at all remarkable if we recall that our eyes are receptors for the brain.

Before there were many words, there were images. Spirits existed everywhere—in the rocks, in the trees, in the sky. Without a highly developed intellectual ability man lived closely in touch with his feelings and sensory impressions. But as language tamed and changed man it moved him further and further away from the pure experience of the moment and into an existence in which intellectualizing about an experience *becomes* the experience. Scuba diving and mountain climbing are experiences; talking and reading about them are likewise experiences, but of a different sort. The same is true when we intellectualize feelings into words, which requires us to abstract and categorize an event or process, and which more or less detaches us from the experience of the moment.

As language developed this process continued unimpeded, and man became more and more separated from his sensory impressions and mystical nature. He became the practical, logical fellow he is today. What we were not aware of until recently is that the totality of our experiences and impressions is related to our ability to be creative and intuitive.

As imagery and spirituality moved further into the background, visionaries lost favor. If one went around talking about hearing God's voice or seeing visions, he was called insane. In the old days you might have been called a saint, depending on what your visions instructed you to do.

Since visions—or the images in one's head—could not easily be intellectualized, they were suppressed. If something could not be seen or shared with others, did it exist? What was it? Demons from a primitive past?

When technology and science displaced religion and myth, the scientists said that every bit of data must have a body of evidence to prove its existence, and must be able to be duplicated by others. But who can duplicate, precisely, the image which floats to mind if you think: Bar Mitzvah. You can share a great deal about that day in your life—the way Uncle Dan and Gus, who hadn't spoken in 10 years, got together and shared too many glasses of wine, or how nervous you were that you would forget some of the words, or how your cousin Ellen met a long-lost relative from Israel and how they now have two-and-a-half kids and live in Northport. Communication is the sharing of images. The more you share, the easier the communication, the greater the empathy.

But at another level, the image and feelings of that day belong to you alone, and all the words in the world will only convey a faint approximation of it. Only you know what really went through your mind.

Or imagine for a moment the most peaceful, restful scene you can. Choose your companions, if you desire. Not one among us will exactly replicate another's corner of nirvana, although many of us will conjure up images that are generally similar.

Imagery is one part of how we think—perhaps the most basic part—and refuses to die, even in our pragmatic world. In the last half-century visualization and imagery in the life of modern-day man were relegated to little more than daydreams, and even there some psychologists tried to say they didn't exist. J. B. Watson, the father of the behaviorism whose ideas held sway in the twenties and thirties, referred to the "fiction of imagery" and put forth instead the concept of subvocal speech: the thought must be uttered silently before the habitual act arises. There was no evidence, he said, for a purely mental experience. We wonder, did Watson ever daydream? Or try out a situation in his head to see how it felt? He must have, for he later left science for advertising and became the father of the Burma Shave sign.

However, those who said behavior could be controlled were to be ever at odds with psychoanalysis, in which imagery played such a large part. Freud used it before he moved into free association, in which a patient in repose talks about whatever comes into his mind. Freud's earlier method was to place his hands on a patient's forehead and exert pressure, telling the patient that when he took his hands away an image would float into his mind, and it would be the key to whatever he was seeking.

Carl Jung dealt heavily in imagination and imagery, for he felt they were tools for acquiring self-knowledge. He recorded his dreams and encouraged his thoughts to drift into fantasies, believing that they held the possibilities and lessons of life. And to him psychic happenings were reality:

> *If a fire burns me, I do not question the reality of the fire, whereas if I am beset by the fear that a ghost will appear, I take refuge behind the thought that it is only an illusion. But just as the first is the psychic image of a physical process whose nature is unknown, so my fear of the ghost is a psychic image from a mental source; it is just as real as the fire, for my fear is as real as the pain caused by the fire.*

Others who would come later kept alive the role of imagination and imagery in psychoanalysis, although it continued to be derided by the behaviorists, who wanted everything to fit neatly onto a chart or graph.

But in the freewheeling sixties when restrictions of all manner were lifted, imagery revived. Perhaps more than many people would like to believe, hallucinogenic drugs, which open a floodgate of imagery, affected the way we began to think and feel about our inner lives, the world, each other and the universality of all things. The first to smoke those funny cigarettes and take little pink sugar lumps were scientists and students, many of whom had formerly rejected the notion that fantasy influenced one's life. The drugs allowed them to get in touch with basic sensory experiences, breaking through rationality and coldly clinical logic. What we are trying to learn now is how to get in touch with these impressions without drugs, and there are some who insist that through the mind's eye it is already possible.

Acid trips were full of images and visions and things which go bump in the night that weren't there when the drugs wore off, but the memory lingered on. In writing, in film, in music and in conversation the influences were felt by all of us, whether or not we directly participated. But before this would happen, imagery would make inroads into hard science.

At some centers, such as Duke University, parapsychological occurrences had been the object of serious study for some years. People who were not mentally disturbed had hallucinations. Studies in sensory deprivation showed that being cut off from hearing, feeling, seeing, smelling and tasting gave rise to visions akin to drug-induced trips. It appears that if the body has no external sensory experience, it creates its own, so great is the need for sensations of some sort. It is what makes us human and what ties us to this world.

For a few years, fasting became popular, and those who tried it for days or weeks found they spent inordinate amounts of time fantasizing about food, which for some later gave way to another kind of awareness.

Some cultures have made use of sensory deprivation as a means to get in touch with imagery. Warriors of certain tribes went into the desert and fasted for days because it was a way to induce dreams or hallucinations that would reveal how they should act in battle, or how their totem poles should be made. Tribes in our Southwest and Mexico continue to use peyote to reach a mystic state that puts them in touch with forces they cannot otherwise reach.

Those who endure deprivations of one sort or another also experience an increase of daydreams, or hallucinations: deep-sea divers, Arctic explorers, prisoners in solitary confinement, desert travellers. Long spans of time in monotonous activity also give rise to diversionary daydreams: truck drivers on night runs often see cars and animals which are not there. Or are they? The folks at NASA who were monitoring Walter Shirra's space flight were very worried for a few minutes when they lost contact with him. Repeated calls went unanswered. Had something happened to the spacecraft, the astronaut or the radio? Shirra was unaware this was going on because he had been . . . ah . . . daydreaming.

Throughout history there have always been people who claimed to see halos or auras enveloping some people; most put them down as crackpots—until a Russian husband and wife team, Semyon and Valentina Kirlian, began photographing these energy emanations. With special equipment they were able to record the electromagnetic field that extends out a few inches around people and plants. When one is calm, the aura is small and pale blue; when one is agitated, it flares to red and orange.

Eastern religion and philosophy, rich with imagery, a belief in a life energy and altered states of consciousness, flourished here at home among those who found Christianity too limiting. Those who could afford to travel—the Beatles and other media stars included—went to the source in India and gave the movement wide publicity. It was celebrated in the songs on our airwaves. Obviously, imagery was an idea whose time had come.

And not quite suddenly, imagery and parapsychology had sneaked past the "hard" scientists (or at least the less doubting of them) because data was being collected on matters that earlier had seemed out of reach. What before had concerned a few believers is now a subject for serious research. But, as St. Thomas Aquinas said centuries ago, all the proofs in the world that a God exists will not convince a skeptic: a leap of faith is necessary. Today research is limiting the areas where blind faith is required.

Visualization is a tool used in vision therapy to improve image memory and thus open the avenues of creativity from the right hemisphere of the brain. With improved visual memory, less effort and time is needed to take in a concept or an event. With words we only comprehend one bit at a time, but visually we can absorb a whole scene. The more you can see, the more you can recall with less effort.

Visualization is the first step to creativity, for in constructing the elements of an event or concept without words we can actually invent new ideas which can later be translated into paintings, statues or words if we must. Einstein translated his visions into formulas.

Visualizing also gives us an opportunity to run through an event before it happens. Our survival depends on it. If we are going to hunt the saber-toothed tiger, it is likely we will imagine what spears to bring along. If we are going to ask the boss for a raise, it is inevitable we will rehearse our lines.

In sports, visualizing the shot beforehand can make a measurable difference to your game. In one famous study, students improved their basketball game substantially by simply imagining that they were sinking basket after basket.

The students who took part were divided into three groups. One group actually practiced making free throws every day for 20 days; another group only practiced twice, on the first and last days. The remaining shooters practiced on the court the first and last day of the survey, but in between they spent 20 minutes every day imagining that they were sinking the ball. They practiced in their heads. They imagined the flight path of the ball as it arched above the rim and plopped into the net. Just as they would have done in real life, if they threw an imaginary shot which missed, they would correct their stance or make some other adjustment until they got the basket.

The students who shot baskets every day improved by 24 percent; the group that played only on the first and last days didn't improve at all. And the students who visualized their shots improved nearly as much as the students who had actually used a basketball. Their shooting ability jumped by 23 percent.

Alan Richardson, the Australian who conducted the study, interviewed the students who took part and concluded that the ability to control the images was the most important factor, not how realistically the scene was imagined. Richardson also concluded that the imagery was most effective if the person *felt* the action taking place as well as simply seeing the pictures. In that way, we suppose, the feeling of successful shooting, of positioning the body, began to be locked into the muscles.

While the techniques taught in vision therapy might certainly improve your darts score, they can also provide a means of helping people understand *visually* how things are in real life. Although it sounds improbable that an architect would have trouble visualizing his designs from different perspectives, it does happen sometimes because he has learned the mechanical rules so well that he gets by relying on them alone. But he won't, in his mind, be able to walk into the kitchen of the house and see how it feels because to him the designs are only pieces of paper with lines on them.

To teach visualizing techniques in therapy a picture will be flashed on a screen and the patient asked to reproduce what he grasped in the twinkling of an eye. He will be asked to take it apart and put it back together again. The individual is asked to see, to relate, to re-create the image. Practice might not make it perfect, but it does make it easier.

In time the person can practice on his own. The architect can try to imagine what a building is like from different perspectives: the back, the sides, above and below. For someone who is able to visualize easily the tasks seem simple, but for someone grounded in the mechanical components of things it takes some doing. Such a person is probably dominated by the left hemisphere of the brain, that side which makes you a whiz at algebra.

To improve visual memory skills, the individual is asked to try to keep the image in his mind's eye without speaking to himself. Ultimately, a person learns to retain many images, and selects from one or another as he sees fit. It's a great help when you have to stop at the grocery store and you don't have your list. Just imagine that you see what you need in your mind's eye.

There are those whose visual memory is so good that they are said to have a photographic memory. They remember by what we call *eidetic images*—the ability to look at a complicated picture, close their eyes and re-create it down to the last detail. Some people can hold such an image for years. The Russian psychologist, A. R. Luria, reported on one individual's ability to see a blackboard full of complicated random numbers, letters and syllables and later rattle them off with ease. He did this by recalling the image precisely as he had seen it and then simply reading the figures.

Creativity

Visualization is a creation of the mind which stays there; art can be the result of that visualization that the creator shares with others, regardless of form: poetry, painting, sculpture, dance, drama. Music, of course, does not begin with pictures, but with sounds instead.

Because the visual arts, drama and dance included, are the attempts of the artist to communicate what his perceptions are, certainly how he creates is dictated by how he sees and perceives the world. His creation does not come out of a vacuum. It is a product not only of his temperament, but also of the temper of the times and the culture in which he lives.

The Japanese, for instance, are renowned for their emotional control. Their homes, furnishings, rock gardens, poetry all reflect this austerity. But within the formal dictates of such rigidly imposed structure are the rumblings of emotions and feelings which run deep and are common to all men. While the Victorian gardens in the West were lush and fanciful, the Japanese kept theirs serene and simple. The poetic form of *haiku* maintains a 17-syllable structure that is spare, clean, and yet provocative:

> Pale moth, if you seek
> only the glitter, it will
> consume before noon.

The Eskimo lives in a world where simplicity of form is dictated by the environment: snow, air, wind and water are basically the only elements with which he deals. When he is out walking, he sees a wash of whitish planes, broken by little else. If his art were to depict only what he saw, it would be similar to our modern minimal painting, no more than subtle shadings of tone, slight form. In response to his barren environment, the Eskimo creates more than just what the eye can see. He paints not only what is present before him, but also what he imagines exists. He paints the ground, and also what is above it and below it, both what he imagines to be there and what he knows is there from previous experience.

The Impressionists (a great many of whom were nearsighted) gave us their personal impression of a scene in color and form, their feelings about the subject rather than a depiction of the scene. To some, such as Matisse, subject matter was of scant importance—what counted was the feeling conveyed to the audience through color. His concern was that the viewer come upon his pictures as one might approach a comfortable old chair.

Vision, then, dictates to a large degree what the artist will create, for he must look to his own perceptions for the message of his mind he wishes to relate to others. As Van Gogh became more and more depressed, his paintings reflected his schizophrenic haze. Gone were the straight lines of bridges and boats; instead lines merged and melded until they were lost in amorphous shapes of color which convey the depths of a man's mind whirling in a starry night.

Perception may, then, either influence style or limit it. The dancer who suppresses vision in the left eye will make little use of the left side of his body; if he choreographs, he will make scant use of left entrances. All the action will be concentrated on the right. He may be aware of this if a critic points it out, and even try to compensate, but as long as vision is unbalanced, this will not come easily.

Keats and Shelley, who shared a time in history as well as a friendship, reflect vast differences in their visual perceptions although both are romantic poets. Keats dealt with subjects which were within a limited visual range, such as the lives and times he saw depicted on a Grecian urn. In "Ode to a Nightingale" he concentrated on senses other than visual:

> I cannot see what flowers are at my feet,
> Nor what soft incense hangs upon the boughs,
> But, in embalmed darkness, guess each sweet
> Wherewith the seasonable month endows
> The grass, the thicket, and the fruit-tree wild;

Shelley, on the other hand, was thought to be farsighted, and dealt with visions far and wide, as in "Ozymandias":

> I met a traveller from an antique land
> Who said: Two vast and trunkless legs of stone
> Stand in the desert. Near them, on the sand,
> Half sunk, a shattered visage lies, whose frown,
> And wrinkled lip, and sneer of cold command,
> Tell that its sculptor well those passions read

Which yet survive, stamped on these lifeless things,
The hand that mocked them and the heart that fed:
And on the pedestal these words appear:
"My name is Ozymandias, king of kings:
Look on my works, ye Mighty, and despair!"
Nothing beside remains. Round the decay
Of that colossal wreck, boundless and bare
The lone and level sands stretch far away.

Although one could say of these two poets that their vision limited them, the beauty of their creations inspires us instead to reflect how it simply influenced them, and look to each for their various perspectives. Likewise, the astigmatism that is believed to have troubled El Greco shaped his paintings. When they are viewed through glasses for a certain degree of astigmatism, they do not appear to be the elongated shapes the rest of us perceive, but look like people of average height and breadth. But that stretched out quality, that surreal thinness El Greco gave his people makes them appear ethereal and mystical, the characteristics for which he is known and admired. It is as if his impaired sight opened the windows to his visionary eye. As linguist S. I. Hayakawa has noted: "The language of vision determines, perhaps even more subtlely and thoroughly than verbal language, the structure of our consciousness."

Healing

One of the most basic and oldest uses of visualization is healing the body. From the beginning, medicine was mostly magic, as the earliest records from Babylonia and Sumer indicate. The medicine man's power stemmed from his ability to visualize the cause of the disease and the cure. Sometimes this would involve potions, dances and chants to combat the evil spirit residing in the body, the imagined cause of the sickness. Today, in some parts of the world, these practices still exist side by side with penicillin, and the doctors who work with primitive tribes frequently see the effectiveness of the ancient ways when our brand of medicine seems to have no effect. Africans in the bush, Canadian Eskimos and the Navajos of the Southwest use forms of healing based on visualization.

The medicine man gets in touch with the evil spirit, puts on a show of force and the spirit dissipates. Among the Eskimos, the shaman journeys in a trance to the bottom of the sea to find the cause of the illness or to ask for help during a storm. The Navajo priest usually instructs helpers in the making of sand paintings, symbols of their gods and the patient's relationship with them. Although the methods vary from tribe to tribe, they have a common base: the ability to imagine that spirits exist—and that they can be called upon.

Religions of the world in technological cultures such as ours still retain that mystic core which depends on visualization: Catholics believe that bread and wine is actually turned into the body and blood of Christ through a process, during Mass, called transubstantiation. All Christians pray to God, and it is permissible to ask for all manner of things, including health for yourself or others. They flock by the thousands to the shrine at Lourdes in France, where an image—or vision—once appeared, and where today crutches and wheelchairs are left behind.

The Christian Scientist believes that disease is a product of the mind, and through praying and by concentrating on the fact that one is healthy, harmony returns to the body. The method of the Rosicrucians, a brotherhood of mystics which goes back to the Renaissance, employs visualizing the ends as a means of reaching them. They do not question the route. They ask that the person to be healed let his consciousness enter in spirit with the sun, allowing its energy to flow through one's being and invigorate it.

Now, although some will find the purely mystical methods of healing unbelievable, we must still be able to account for the unexplainable, even in the rigorously scientific world of modern medical research. Consider the lowly placebo.

When screening new drugs a researcher must be positive that the effects he gets are caused by the medicine in question and not by some extraneous factor, such as nutrition, genetics or the phase of the moon. In sophisticated drug experiments a duplicate of the pill being tested will be given to some of the people; but these pills will be only copies, a dummy with no possible therapeutic value. Called placebos, they are included against the unlikely chance that some people are recovering due to an unexpected quality of the disease, or against the more outlandish possibility that they are getting well simply because someone in a white lab coat told them they would.

That a suggestion—an image—could produce a physiological change in the system of chemicals we call our bodies was patently ridiculous, but researchers being skeptics and recognizing the existence of spontaneous remission, they needed this trick pill to sort out the unexpected. A rich harvest they have had.

In one study patients who had been hospitalized with bleeding ulcers showed a 70 percent improvement over a period of a year when they were given an injection of distilled water and assured that it was a new medicine that would cure them.

The treatment of warts is sometimes based on the placebo effect, even though they are caused by a virus. Patients have had warts painted with inert dyes, placed pennies over them, and even rubbed raw potatoes on them. One doctor with a high rate of success merely tells his patients the warts will go away.

As we have said all along, changes in the environment can well be all in a person's mind, which in turn produces a change in the body. As the brain stimulates itself—one neuron sending a message to another —the brain provides its own environment. There is an environment outside the body: it's where we live. There is an environment inside the body: it's where the brain resides. And just as the weather outside tells us how to dress, the body is always sending messages from all points to the brain, and the brain sends messages back.

Among the members of an Australian tribe, the Murngin, the power of suggestion appears to have life and death consequences. If a Murngin is told that his spirit has been stolen, and others in the tribe learn of his fate, he dies within several days. When the body is examined no disease is found. But if a Murngin near death is told that the spell has been broken and his soul has come back home, he frequently recovers. It is speculated that the death may be caused by excessive adrenaline produced by the stress of believing one is about to die. You see, the Murngin *knows* the curse works.

Yogis likewise astounded Western science because they could control body functions to a degree for which there appeared to be no reasonable explanation. It has been routinely believed that we had no control over our involuntary autonomic system, which regulates heart beat, blood pressure, digestion and the like. Shortly after the turn of the century information began to pile up in the United States and Germany that such was not the case. Experiments were proving otherwise: if we choose to, we can control body processes to a measurable degree.

An American physiologist, Edmund Jacobson, began experimenting with the effects of internal suggestion. He had people imagine that they were running. Small—but measurable—muscular contractions took place, of the same type that would have occurred if the subjects had actually been running. A change in the mental environment of the brain had effected a change in the muscles of the body. It should be pointed

out that Jacobson's studies were confined to the muscles under voluntary control, the same ones that would have been in motion if the person actually had been running.

But the involuntary muscle system would also have been under
stimulation of some sort, and similarly would have caused a change in
the organism, as Dr. Mike Samuels and his wife, Nancy, explain in *Seeing with the Mind's Eye:*

> *. . . anatomists have also long been aware of pathways between
> the cerebral cortex, where images are stored, and the autonomic
> nervous system which controls the so-called involuntary muscles.
> The autonomic nervous system controls sweating, blood vessel ex-
> pansion and contraction, blood pressure, blushing and goosepim-
> pling, the rate and force of heart contraction, respiratory rate, dry-
> ness of mouth, bowel motility and smooth muscle tension. There
> are also pathways between the autonomic nervous system and the
> pituitary and adrenal cortex. The pituitary gland secretes hormones
> which regulate the rate of secretion of other glands; especially the
> thyroid, sex and adrenal glands. The adrenal glands secrete ste-
> roids, which regulate metabolic processes, and epinephrine, which
> causes the 'fight or flight' reaction. Through these pathways, an
> image held in the mind can literally affect every cell in the body.*

What we know as emotions can be seen as an intermediate part
of a chain reaction that involves vast and elaborate interactions, starting in the eyes and quickly encompassing both our voluntary and involuntary systems. When visual images—those untouchable, unmea-
surable, yet undeniably real optic events—somehow initiate within us a
noticeable physical reaction, we often label the process *emotion*. The
word *emotion* is simply a device we use to explain those situations when
a visualization and the energy it involves chemically activate our brain,
which in turn impinges physically on our body. This may sound confusing to those who aren't familiar with physiology, but you undoubtedly
recognize the physical power of a visual image when you find yourself
nauseated at the thought of an impending dinner with your disapproving
in-laws.

All these processes do not turn on and off by themselves; the
master switch in the brain has been touched by the image in your
mind. A German psychiatrist and neurologist, J. H. Schultz, was the
first to demonstrate precisely to what extent we could voluntarily control
our bodily functions. In the twenties and thirties he developed *autogenic*

therapy, a treatment which Schultz claimed can be used for whatever ails you. Dr. Schultz would ask his patients to sit or lie down comfortably, close their eyes, tell them to imagine they were in mental contact with that part of the body they wished to effect, have them repeat a given formula—in words or images—and ask them to be casual about the whole process.

For instance, someone who is plagued by cold feet might think how warm his feet felt. It worked. Cold feet turned warm. When measured systematically, the autosuggestion was shown to increase blood flow, relax blood vessels, and promote healing. His method seems to say that we can be as healthy as we wish ourselves to be. It doesn't sound unlike the beliefs of the Christian Scientists and Rosicrucians.

Schultz also realized that the relaxed state of consciousness in which his patients did the exercises could also be used to get at buried feelings or come to a new level of self-awareness and knowledge. He developed meditative exercises to question the inner self about those secrets of the heart which you don't consciously admit to.

Autogenic training became popular in Europe, where its results were extensively documented with thousands of case studies. Among the bodily functions altered by it are temperature, blood sugar, white blood cell count, blood pressure, heart and breathing rate, brain waves and thyroid secretion. The training not only affects the body in general, but also treats the specific complaints. In combination with drugs and surgery, the technique has been used with varying degrees of success to treat just about everything: ulcers, hemorrhoids, constipation, obesity, heart conditions, headaches, blood pressure, arthritis, back pain, angina and gall bladder attacks.

The medical profession in Europe more or less accepted that autogenic training can and does work, possibly because one of their own did the work, but it was not taken seriously in America until the late sixties when we discovered we could control the electrical quality of our brainwaves. We learned how to encourage our nightly drift into the euphoria of alpha, a relaxed state characterized by the absence of visual activity. With biofeedback equipment monitoring our physiological responses, we learned that it was possible to get rid of migraines and even teach an epileptic how to spot the abnormal brainwaves that precede a seizure and send it away. It turned out that the control we have is so sophisticated that man can at will fire only one or two specific neurons out of the hundreds of millions of which he is made.

Dr. Neil Miller, a pioneer biofeedback researcher, demonstrated that some animals could even be taught to alter the thickness of their stomach walls and learn such fine control of their blood vessels that they could turn one ear white and the other brilliant pink. Naturally, he reasoned, that if animals could be taught such control, certainly so could humans.

What the Zen and Yoga masters had long demonstrated was now proven to the satisfaction of the scientific community. Researchers who might have scoffed at the claims put forth by such diverse practices as self-hypnosis, psychic healing, yoga and the methods of modern-day mind-control systems such as Arica and Silva Mind Control could no longer do so.

Biofeedback equipment monitors the subject's bodily activity so that he can see the energy as it is registered by a needle. By making an effort to control that needle, even if the subject does not understand precisely how he is able to do it, he produces the evidence that his mind and his body are one.

One amusing anecdote reported by Elmer and Alyce Green of the Menninger Foundation in *Beyond Biofeedback* is a good example of how precise visualization can be. A university professor was trying to warm one hand and cool the other, and although he had raised the temperature of one hand by as much as seven degrees in four minutes, he was having difficulty in getting the other hand to cool down. Suddenly, after three minutes, the temperature gauge attached to the warm hand began to register a lower temperature and dropped five degrees in a minute.

Dr. Green wanted to know how the professor accomplished this with such speed. "He laughed and said that he had goofed at first. When nothing happened after a couple of minutes, he realized that his visualization was wrong. His refrigerator door had a hinge on the left, and he always opened the door with his left hand and took out the ice-cube tray with his right hand. In his imagination he had tried to put his left hand on the ice cubes, but his body knew better than that and wouldn't respond. After he corrected the visualization the temperature difference between the two hands changed rapidly."

It appears that not only is it possible to control the internal workings of the system, we can even learn how to alter its physical appearance. At a few centers throughout the country, including the University of Houston, experiments with women who wish to enlarge the size of their breasts are working. They simply imagine their breasts are already larger. Sometimes hypnotic suggestion is used, sometimes only visualization techniques. In one study the women were told to visualize a warm towel over their breasts and then a heat lamp over that, and to practice as often as they wished.

As reported in the *American Journal of Clinical Hypnosis* last year, breast size in one study increased to the point where almost half of the 22 women participating found it necessary to buy a larger bra. At the same time many of them actually lost weight, so the increase in chest circumference could not be attributed to extra pounds. The average increase in breast measurement was slightly under one-and-a-half inches in one study, two inches in another.

According to Sidney Petrie of the New York Institute for Hypnotherapy, "If the mind perceives something as happening, it tends to make organic changes happen." The researchers have said they believe the change occurs because of increased blood flow within the breasts. Although it is generally thought that breast developing devices advertised at the back of women's magazines are not as effective as the copy claims, there are those impressive "after" photographs. The women who do succeed may do so because they believe in the gadget.

In 1965 a radiologist in Fort Worth began using visualization in combination with conventional therapy to treat cancer patients, and he reports encouraging results. Dr. Carl Simonton became interested in trying something different when he contemplated the many patients who were considered terminal, yet who recovered. He believed it was due to a positive attitude towards life and the desire to get well. He had observed that patients often lived long enough to witness a special event they were looking forward to—a reunion with a lost member of the family or a granddaughter's graduation from law school.

It is Dr. Simonton's thesis that we all contract some type of cancer during our lives, but our immunological system takes care of it before the cancer spreads. He set out to find a way to encourage the patient to turn on his immunological system. Dr. Simonton, and his wife Stephanie, decided to try a therapy consisting of visualization of the body curing itself and group discussions among the patients.

The cancer victim is taught to go into deep relaxation, then to imagine a peaceful scene, and then to see his cancer in his mind's eye and to picture an army of healthy white cells attacking the tumorous growth and carrying off the malignant ones—which also had been weakened by the patient's continued traditional therapy.

The patients learn how their immune system works, look at their own X rays and pictures of tumors healing. In group discussions many uncover their perhaps hidden fears about becoming well. If a lonely widow is ill with cancer, her children will visit her more often; but will they come on Sundays if she is healthy? The problem in life is that the antidote for some real or imagined grievance is often much worse than the emotion causing it.

Although the patient usually begins by trying to construct an image of the tumor, obviously this image in the mind's eye is infinitely subjective. One man, Bob Gilley, responded by making a game of the exercise. In his mind the cancer was a vicious animal, sometimes a snake. The white blood cells were visualized as healthy white husky dogs, ripping the snake apart. Naturally the good dogs won. After the battle they would lick up the residue and clean his abdominal cavity.

Gilley did the exercise three times a day, for 10 to 15 minutes. His chances of survival had been estimated at 30 percent. After six weeks of imagery therapy his tumor had shrunk by 75 percent, and two months later there was not a trace of the disease left in his body. Of course, by no means do all individuals have the sort of success that he had.

Although the Simontons are still compiling data on their work, approximately 18 percent of the 150 patients who have been treated at their Cancer Counseling and Research Center in Fort Worth since 1972 show no incidence of the disease. All had been diagnosed as terminal. A full 40 percent are leading active lives.

Imagery as a tool is available to all of us, whether we are physically sick or not. Through imagination (call it daydreaming if you must) we can become aware of our feelings and attitudes of which we may not normally be conscious. It's those secrets we keep from ourselves that often govern our lives.

Free-floating imagery lets us look beyond the immediacy of a sickness and examine the negative feelings which may be the heart of the matter. Sickness always changes the situation: a lonely wife buys her husband's attention if she has to go to the hospital; a person unhappy with his job finds he doesn't have to go to work when he's sick with a cold which keeps him in bed; an alcoholic doesn't have to deal with feelings of failure. We are not saying, of course, that all illnesses are caused by emotional queasiness of one sort or another, but we do recognize that for every emotional action there is a physical response, and for every physical action there is a psychological counterpart as well.

The Russians, who appear to be ahead of us in research in the parapsychological, report that others can influence much more than your emotions—they can reach right down to your blood cells. When the researchers directed positive emotions and happy feelings toward their subjects, the number of white blood cells, which are the main-line defense in the body, rose dramatically. Negative thoughts had the opposite effect. It makes a skeptic wonder about the value of prayer.

You might be suffering through a cold as you read this and have difficulty imagining that it was caused by anything other than your husband's sneezing, or the fact that last week you waited 15 minutes for the bus in the rain. But haven't you done that before and not gotten sick? This time your body wasn't able to marshal enough defenses to suppress the illness. We recognize that nutrition and other factors come into play when one gets sick; but there are always some people who seem to do everything possible to take care of their physical needs—and always catch the flu when it's going around.

Knowing how to relax and erase the cares of the day might be one way we can help ourselves to health. Dr. Herbert Benson of Harvard Medical School studied the soothing effects of transcendental meditation and determined that we could employ a similar method for psychological and physical benefits. The question whether the mind and body could affect each other was hardly considered: Of course they could.

By instructing people to rest quietly in a dim place, close their eyes and repeat the number *one,* or to concentrate on another sound, a phrase that was repeated again and again, telling them not to worry about how well they were doing, Dr. Benson could elicit several physiological changes which he has termed the relaxation response. After 12 minutes of relaxation oxygen consumption was down, carbon-dioxide production decreased, breathing was slowed. Eventually blood pressure lowers, and there are decreased waste products in the blood.

Dr. Benson's work showed that there are indeed ways the yogis could have gained such control over their bodies when they instructed their minds what their bodies were to do. There are stories of masters in the mountains of Tibet who can sit almost naked in the snow—and melt the snow around them. And there are some who believe that pain, incredible though it may seem, is a *learned* response. (However, it should be pointed out that it is also a defense mechanism to let you know when you are burning your hand. If a child felt no pain why should he move his hand out of the flame?)

We have concentrated on the visualization techniques that are finding their way into traditional medicine. The premise has been to show that these techniques of the mind indeed have an effect on the body, and that these changes can be measured in the laboratory.

But there is a whole group of people who have never doubted that imagination—call it meditation, prayer, relaxation, self-hypnosis or any name you like—can cure: faith healers. The President's sister, Ruth Carter Stapleton, is one; so is Reverend Ike. These healers exist in Spanish Harlem; they thrive in the Bible Belt. Many of them believe that you will get whatever it is you want as long as the desire is deep enough and the faith is absolute. It may be that simply by imagining what you want, the willing spirit controls the unwitting flesh.

The faith healers' results have been derided by the medical profession, which usually does not welcome therapies other than their own. The cures, by their thinking, seem illogical and therefore improbable. Admittedly, the claims often put forth seem incongruous and unreal. But then so do a lot of things.

Researchers in the laboratories and doctors in the clinics are coming up with much the same results by approaching the problem somewhat differently. They ask not that the patient believe in the healer but in his own ability to facilitate the healing force: The Chinese call it *chi,* the Indians, *prana* or *kundalini,* the Sufis, *baraka.* In the fifties Wilhelm Reich called it *orgone* energy. In *Star Wars* it's called The Force.

In any event, if you believe in such a thing, its effects depend on your own desire and ability to call upon it and make friends with it. Remember, it's all in your mind's eye.

One way to succeed is to imagine the final result and stay with the good feelings associated with that. Use imagination, and the means should take care of themselves. This will certainly save you from a lot of day-to-day aggravation when what you want is taking longer than you would like. "Time is no longer a hindrance, but a means of making actual what is potential" is a line from the *I Ching,* or *Book of Changes,* which was written in the century before Confucius.

4
Color–Fact and Fantasy

We cannot lose what really belongs to us, even if we throw it away. Therefore, we need have no anxiety. All that need concern us is that we should remain true to our own natures and not listen to others.

Remember when you were a child and you shut your eyes and the colors of the rainbow would switch on—sometimes to the point where you couldn't get to sleep because the light show wasn't over yet? Or how you saw pink and white stars that came and went in a twinkling when you rubbed your eyes?

But when we grow up these vivid flashes disappear from our nights, and we no longer think about them except once in a while when recalling the delights of childhood. When asked, many an adult will say: I don't see them anymore. Along the trip from youth to adulthood, something happened which switched them off.

These color visualizations are the stuff upon which an ancient form of healing is based, and although color therapy smacks of the occult, today some serious researchers, most of whom would scoff at matters psychic, are coming up with seemingly amazing results. However, it is true that many color therapists are tied to astrology, numerology and such, and their claims tend to sound unbelievable. Some years ago, the fantastic results reported by a few color therapists led to legal action against them. As a result, most work in this area is being done in England and New Zealand and is known here largely through word of mouth.

Color is such an ineluctable part of our lives it is hard to imagine that it can have any effect other than to please or irritate. And therein lies the clue—all of us are aware that there are some colors we like and some we don't, some make us feel calm, others are energizing. And if, as we have been saying all along, for each psychological event there is a physiological reaction, the premise that color might influence our well-being does not sound so wild after all.

Just as the connection between vision and comprehension never died in language, and we continue to say things such as "I see what you mean," so is color entwined in our spoken communication. We *see red* when we are angry, become *green with envy, feel blue* or are *in the pink* and have a *rosy future.* The phrases are apt for the feeling each color projects, just as music sends out various vibrations of mood.

In fact, color and musical tone are thought by some to be different forms of vibrating frequencies of energy. At a certain octave, the wave frequency is transmitted as sound; at a higher frequency the energy is transmitted as light and color.

As we prefer Beethoven one day and Stravinsky another, as we need to run and need to rest, so do we choose our colors. We don't have to think about it; we just feel drawn to one piece of music or hue of the rainbow. One season you might be attracted to brown and fill up your closet with items in every shade of it; next winter they all seem drab and depressing, and brighter shades appeal. Color healers would tell you that the psychological lift we get from your sunny new apparel is not a frivolous waste of money.

If we consider light a source of energy, nutrition as it were, it is reasonable to assume that each kind of light—each color—will have a different nutritive effect. Red meat has different nutrients from white fish, even though both are sources of protein. Generally, foods of a certain color tend to have the same vitamins: reddish foods (such as meat and beets) frequently are high sources of the B vitamins; yellow-green foods (lemons, most greens) are rich in Vitamin C.

At this stage of knowledge our concept of color is a combination of two theories, and the reality is probably somewhere in between. Einstein proposed that light is a form of energy and radiates in a narrow beam, travelling through space as an impulse of packets of energy. But light also acts like a wave, with a crest and a trough. When two beams of light hit each other crest to crest, their brightness increases, and when a crest of one wave touches a trough of another, the brightness is diminished.

Although it is generally believed that the two theories complement one another, light remains a mystery even to the physicists, because sometimes it behaves like a fast-flying particle and at other times like a wave. We do know that no matter what form it assumes it travels at the speed of 186,000 miles per second, which is a whole lot faster than any of us can imagine. That is one of those facts which at this stage of our evolution we accept without fully comprehending; we memorize without feeling how it works.

Sir Isaac Newton passed light through a prism and a single white beam was dispersed into several colors—red, orange, yellow, green, blue, indigo and violet. He attempted to relate them to the seven notes in an octave, and while critics derided that connection as mystical nonsense, today there are some who would say he was right.

Sound, in fact, has an effect on our perception of color. Low-pitched sounds tend to make color appear to deepen: red moves toward blue, orange appears more red. The opposite is true of high-pitched tones, which make colors seem lighter. Sound has been found to affect the sensitivity of the eye's rods—the more sound, the less sensitive the rods. It's a happy occurrence, because the rods do their work at night, when the world usually turns down the volume. When noise increases what can be seen on the outer boundaries of the retina grows dim.

On the other hand, sound increases the sensitivity of the cones, which operate during daylight when the volume is usually greater. Hearing and vision are interlocked, for both the eye and the ear respond to waves of energy.

The tone that we hear depends upon the wavelength of the sound energy that strikes our ear drums—the sound of a French horn, Ella Fitzgerald, garbage trucks at 6 a.m.

The colors that we see are different because light has different wavelengths: a different size space between each crest, if we wish to think of light rays as ocean waves. Red has the longest wavelength, violet the shortest, and we perceive the different wavelengths as different colors, with our eyes tuned in to seven basic differences.

But what makes some apples red, some green, the Aegean Sea turquoise, the grass green, the sky blue? When light strikes an object, such as an apple, that object acquires the color we see by reflecting that color. All the other colors are absorbed, and the one single wavelength which bounces back and into our eyes is the color that our brain assigns to the object. Certain objects reflect similar types of light, even combinations of tiny light variations, and we group them under an energy label: green.

White light, white underwear, white anything is an equal combination of all the colors in the rainbow mixed together, scattered and reflected back in the energy band we call white. Conversely, when all the colors are absorbed and are not reflected back, we call an object black.

The light frequency sends a particular message through our visual apparatus, and we put the color together in our mind's eyes, making sense out of particular frequencies that stimulate neural impulses one way for red, another for purple. The apple's red, then, exists in your mind's eye—and not in the apple.

We have touched upon how light affects us in more ways than simply allowing us to see. Later we will discuss how anything other than the full spectrum of natural sunlight has been shown to produce abnormalities. Full-spectrum light on the eyes appears to affect the functioning of the pituitary and pineal glands, which control the production of hormones and have a great deal to do with how we feel.

Intuitively we know that sunlight (which contains all the colors of the spectrum) imbues us with a sense of well-being. Pliny stated that the secret of Rome's becoming the mightiest of nations had to do with the fact that its citizens frequently sunbathed on the roofs of their houses. In modern times it has been noted that when we live in areas deprived of sun, our skins take on a pallor generally considered to be unhealthy; in the sunlight, pain, fever and chills dissipate, infections, acne and ulcers heal more quickly. Several studies attest to the fact that being in the darkness decreases the red cell count of the blood, and light increases it. In either event the blood tends to right itself when the light is stabilized, that is, when we are sometimes in the dark and sometimes in the light.

In addition to the effects of brightness, it has been shown that certain colors can affect us physiologically. In some circumstances it appears that color can be beneficial and have healing properties. When an infant is born with jaundice, giving the skin a sickly yellowish cast, a blue light shining in the nursery may reverse the condition, depending on the cause of the jaundice. The yellow apparent in the skin is often the result of a high bilirubin level in the blood. Bilirubin is a yellowish substance formed when the body breaks down hemoglobin, the red cell material that transports oxygen throughout the body. If the level of bilirubin is too high, brain damage and cerebral palsy may result. Premature infants often have livers which are not equipped to deal with this problem, and jaundice is the result. Infants born of parents with incompatible blood are the most susceptible. Previously the only treatment was a complete transfusion. All the blood was taken out and then replaced, a treatment which obviously endangered the infant.

In 1958 an English doctor, Dr. Richard Cremer, accidentally discovered that the bilirubin level could be corrected with artificial blue light in the nursery for eight hours a day for five or six days. Today, the blue-light treatment is replacing the need for some transfusions. In the case of infants with parents whose blood is incompatible, the initial transfusion may still be necessary, but the need for additional ones is diminished. At some medical centers, daylight white fluorescent, which more nearly emulates the full spectrum of light from the sun, has been found to work nearly as well as blue lights and is the treatment used.

Recently, there have been some indications that artificial colors in food can cause irritability. As a result, allergist Dr. Ben Feingold suggests carefully scrutinizing food eaten by hyperactive children. It appears that the ingested color reacts with certain wavelengths of light in the environment and in some children produces adverse reactions.

In like fashion certain drugs, such as the tetracyclines, make some people burn more readily in the sun. As a result the dosage required may be different if you are wintering in sunny climes rather than the north woods.

The profound effect of sunlight on human beings can be appreciated from the fact that its total absence can make a woman temporarily infertile. It happens near the Arctic Circle during the dark winter days when their land is unrelieved by sunlight.

But even an ordinary light bulb can affect a woman's cycle. This was demonstrated by two Boston doctors some years ago when they treated 25 women with irregular menstrual cycles by asking them to keep their bedroom lights burning all night from the 14th to the 16th day of their cycle, the time when they would probably be ovulating. All but two of the women became regular. It is assumed that the light passing through the closed eyelids entered the body and stimulated the brain.

If light is somehow related to behavior and the female's ability to conceive, might it also influence the sex of her offspring? Well, it appears to do so in chinchillas. In 1970 statistics compiled over five years by more than 2,000 ranchers demonstrated that the ratio of females to males could be altered by the color of light under which the mothers lived. Chinchillas, when bred under ordinary incandescent lighting—such as plain light bulbs—have litters averaging 60 to 75 percent male; when the bulbs were changed to "daylight" bulbs—which have a transparent bluish glass—the ratio of females to males reverses.*

---

* Recent studies indicate that we may have found the answer for the world's food supply. When cattle are given 16-hour days (with artificial light) they achieve greater girth and weight. The same is apparently true for chickens.

Although we continue to think of blue for boys, this study shows that perhaps it should be the other way around. Now we are not suggesting that if you want a boy you replace your bedroom bulbs with soft, pink "romantic" bulbs; in fact, pink light produces irritability and tension when it is installed in offices to provide a softer feeling, according to one of the world's leading light experts, John Ott. His studies, and those of others, are enumerated in his book, *Health & Light.*

The breeding of mink is particularly fascinating. Mink, normally a somewhat nasty lot requiring handlers to wear heavy gloves, became positively fierce when kept under deep pink glass through which the sunlight filtered. But kept under blue plastic, they became friendly and docile and could be handled with bare hands.

The same friendliness obviously extended to one another, for all the females in one trial became pregnant under blue light, and all of the males were found to be "working," to use the vernacular of the mink industry. Under pink the statistics went the other way. All females had to be injected with the serum of pregnant mares, which helps matters along, and yet only 87 percent became pregnant. The statistic does not please mink breeders. Ninety percent of the males were "non-working." Makes one wonder about those pink-tinted lenses which are popular today. In one informal personality survey, three college students out of 300 were found to be "disturbed." All three wore pink lenses.

In laboratory tests, pink fluorescent lighting kept on for 12 hours a day over a period of six months caused the tails of mice gradually to slough off. This group also had the lowest survival rate as compared to mice kept under various types of fluorescent. Survival was highest under daylight which nearly approximates the full spectrum of sunlight. Research that has not been widely publicized has shown that limited spectrum fluorescent lighting—cool white, for instance—can have a deleterious effect on health, both mental and physical. (This will be discussed at greater length in Chapter 7.)

Plant life is similarly affected by color. Ott began his study of light while he was developing the art of time-lapse photography, in which a plant seems to bloom in a matter of minutes. He was having a great deal of difficulty in filming the growth of a pumpkin.

A pumpkin has both male and female flowers, and they must cross-pollinate to reproduce a baby pumpkin. The first year on the project, all the female flowers dropped off while the males were doing fine. Ott decided to try again the following year, but he replaced a burned-out fluorescent tube with a daylight white tube. Daylight white is slightly bluish in color; it makes ladies' lipstick look ghoulish and purple—and it turned out to make female pumpkin flowers blossom. Alas, the males withered on the vine. Undaunted, Ott sent out a call to friends in Florida who found a male pumpkin flower in bloom. It was flown up to Chicago where the arranged marriage produced a baby pumpkin, who went on to have a starring role in Walt Disney's *Secrets of Life.*

Generally, long-wave light (red, orange) appears to accelerate plant growth, while short-wave (green, blue, violet) retards it. Plants that bloom during the long days of summer sunlight, such as stock, are found to grow tallest when exposed to orange-red light; they do not bloom at all under yellow, green or blue light, although they do produce heavy foliage. Morning glories, however, which open in the dark before dawn, do best under blue and fail under red. As with humans, it's all a matter of personal preference.

Fish that spend their lives in aquariums thrive if a blacklight, which emits ultraviolet waves that are safe and good for us, is kept on at least part of the day. It not only prevents a disease known as "pop eye" but also puts a stop to the fin-nipping that is common among fish. Some fish cannot be kept alive in captivity without the added blacklight.

Although discos often use this kind of lighting for effect rather than health (it makes white glow in the dark), those who frequent them may be doing themselves a bit of good. At one Chicago seafood restaurant, according to Ott, the ultraviolet light was added many years ago for special effects. When the owner was queried about the health of the employees he discovered that they generally got along extremely well, were seldom ill, and that he had the same crew of waiters who had been there when the lights were installed—18 years before. Makes you wonder.

Although most of us are aware that there are some colors we are attracted to and some we shun, is there evidence that would prove color elicits physiological changes which can be measured? That was the question Robert Gerard set out to answer a few years ago when he was working on his doctorate at the University of California at Los Angeles.

Does red arouse? Does blue calm? Do they cause responses in the nervous system?

Gerard's research confirmed intuition: red does excite, blue does soothe. He did detailed studies of blood pressure, the conductivity of the palm that indicates the arousal of the autonomic nervous system, breathing, heartbeat, muscle activity, eyeblinks and brain waves. He also asked the subjects how they felt.

The more anxious the subjects, the more red disturbed them. Blood pressure, eye blinks, palm conductivity and breathing rate went up under red, down under blue. No difference was found in heartbeat, but in brain-wave activity, while the brain showed an immediate response to red, white and blue (the only colors used in the experiments), after 10 minutes the activity remained consistently greater for red than for blue. In all of the tests, white was found to elicit a response similar to red.

Faber Birren, the noted color authority, suggests in *Color Psychology and Color Therapy* that perhaps the calming effect of blue could be used to alleviate hypertension. It may also act as a tranquilizer and be helpful in treating eye irritations and insomnia. Red might turn your bedroom into a nest of passion, but blue will help you to sleep.

Restaurateurs for years have known that vivid red tends to make diners outgoing and expansive, and they use it in the decor of many posh eating places. How many more times have you seen red goblets, red tablecloths and red-flocked wallpaper than, say, yellow or green in restaurants? Yellow, in fact, is thought to depress appetites, so unless you're battling the bulge it's best to keep it out of the dining room.

Darell Boyd Harmon, an educational researcher, found that the soft, warm colors in the red family, such as peach, tan and the light emitted from warm fluorescence are conducive to intellectual pursuits and would be good choices in schools, libraries and any place where studying is to be done.

Soft, cool colors, such as green, blue-green and the light from cool fluorescence are favorable for movement and would be ideal in a gymnasium. However, the deeper, brighter blues have a tendency to orient a person inward, just as deep and vivid red tones energize. The knowledge that red impels people to action has been put to use by some school coaches: They have the home team's locker room painted red, the visitors', a low-energy blue.

The tendency today, however, is to disregard the color and concentrate solely on assuring adequate lightness and brightness, and while these are important, there are other considerations. The brightness needed to combat the dark walls that decorators make popular every other decade may impede your concentration. Think how often you close your eyes to solve a complex problem or comprehend difficult material; you are blocking out all visual stimulation which may be distracting. Color should be directed to help your concentration, not fight against it.

Sometimes closing your eyes isn't enough. In experiments some years ago, when the faces and necks of subjects were illuminated and their eyes tightly sealed, they tended to move their outstretched arms toward the light, if it was red, and away from it if blue. The same phenomenon is said to have been observed in blind persons. This shows that color affects us even when absorbed through the skin.

One researcher claims that the kind of light which enters the body through the colored pupils of our eyes has something to do with personality. Morgan Worthy, a Georgia State University psychologist, concludes that light and dark eyes let through varying amounts of short and long wavelengths, which in turn regulate our psychological and physical state.

Dark eyes have a lot of pigment and block more short-wave light than long-wave light, and it appears that long waves more frequently activate the pineal and hypothalamus glands. Light eyes let through more short-wave light.

Worthy's observations over the last several years have led him to conclude that light-eyed people and animals tend to do better at detached analytical tasks (that cool blue again), while dark-eyed creatures lean toward hot-blooded emotional reactions. It is worth pointing out that these qualities sound like those associated with red, and since red is the longest wavelength in the spectrum, it appears that red would be activating the glands. What you feel may be what is happening inside.

He describes the two types of individuals as self-paced (light-eyed) and reactive (dark-eyed). Self-paced tasks are those in which the individual has a certain amount of control, because they can be performed in his own time. Hitting a golf ball and writing are self-paced, because they can be done when an individual chooses. Among animals, self-paced tasks are those demanding long periods of patience, such as when a cat waits for a mouse to appear. Reactive tasks, on the other hand, require an instant response to the actions of another, such as when a baseball batter lays into a fast pitch.

His initial interest in the relation between eye color and performance of specific abilities was sparked by the observation that black athletes (most of whom have dark eyes) seem to excel at reactive tasks such as blocking a football pass, while quarterbacks, who pace their movements to their own analysis of the situation, tend to have light eyes. He discounted racial discrimination in sports as a reason for this when he observed that the "greater the percentage of blacks playing a position, the darker the eyes of the whites who play that same position."

Among dogs, Worthy found that those bred for the reactive life of a pet or watchdog have dark eyes, while those bred for self-paced hunting ability, such as setters and pointers, tend to have lighter eyes.

Worthy carefully notes in *Eye Color, Sex and Race* that eye color does not help or hinder a person in carrying out a specific act, but that there appears to be a genetic link between eye color and what a person does best. He points out that his conclusions apply to groups rather than individuals, and that neither blue eyes or brown eyes are to be preferred or are more desirable. Beauty may be in the eye of the beholder, but one may be attracted to more than simply blue eyes.

Color Therapy

The use of color in therapy has been attempted in one form or another since the ancient Egyptians. The healers divined which color the patient was deficient in and put him in a room of that color. Colored gems were also used, and could either be worn, held, or used to treat water: you soak the gem in the water, which charges it with the color of the gem, and then drink it. Pythagoras experimented with this type of therapy, basing his methods on the notion that color could be "fed" through the eyes.

Color therapists today generally believe that when the body is in balance it filters out of white light the colors that are needed. When something's amiss, hues applied in a variety of ways, even wearing a light blue sweater on a day you have a sore throat, will be salubrious. Green, for instance, is thought to build muscle and tissue, and likewise, they attest, eating green foods will also help. Considering that green vegetables are a rich source of vitamins and minerals, needed to build strong tissues, the color therapists have a point there. Unfortunately, medical researchers have not yet taken this work seriously enough to provide us with sufficient data to sort out the facts.

Color Treatment for Optical Problems

There is some work being done today to use colors in treating optical distortions such as nearsightedness and farsightedness. In normal vision the individual sees red and blue equally clearly. The myopic patient sees the red end of the spectrum more easily than the blue because the red wavelength is refracted so that it falls closer to his retina. Blue falls closer to the retina in the farsighted individual. In this treatment a nearsighted person looks at charts through red filters and gradually progresses to the blue end of the spectrum. The opposite is used for the farsighted individual.

There is also a new treatment for color blindness. A single pink contact lens is prescribed for one eye only. This seems to allow the individual to discern colors more easily.

Intuition tells us that color affects us psychologically. One researcher who has studied the connection for many years has, in fact, devised a psychological test which can be compared to an inkblot test. Dr. Max Luscher, a professor of psychology at Basel University in Switzerland, found that the colors you preferred out of a packet of eight would reveal mood, tendencies and aspirations at the time you took the test.

Color is thought to reach us in feeling and is not something which we easily verbalize. The artist whose palette is dark is probably depressed; when spirits lift, so will the colors. But the colors themselves may have something to do with the process, nurturing the gloomy or good feelings along.

part two

5
Is Vision Inherited or Is It Learned?

The fate of fire depends on wood; as long as there is wood below, the fire burns above. It is the same in human life; there is in man likewise a fate that lends power to his life.

Once upon a time it was thought that we got to be who we are almost entirely through heredity. By this logic, intelligent, thrifty, loyal and wise parents would always produce children who were intelligent, thrifty, loyal and wise. It was in the genes. Conversely, children of a beggarman or thief didn't stand much of a chance to be other than outcasts like their parents.

It didn't always work that way. Charles Dickens's father was something of a scoundrel, and Joan of Arc was born of shepherds. Probably your own experience includes someone who seemingly didn't turn out like his parents. But consider this: Dickens went on to write about characters like his father (as all writers use their own experiences for material) and Joan of Arc, though she became counselor to a king, never lost her peasant ways.

During this century one school of psychologists codified what a lot of people already sensed: The experiences of a lifetime influence what a child grows up to be. Their theory was that a child was more or less a blank slate upon which certain behavioral patterns could be inscribed through conditioning.

The idea was hardly new. It harks back to the concepts of the seventeenth-century English philosopher John Locke, who postulated that a child's mind was a *tabula rasa,* without preconceptions. Although the theory coincided neatly with the egalitarian spirit of the times, the

107

rigid class structure prevented it from becoming much more than parlor talk among the intelligentsia, and it remained for the twentieth-century behaviorists to attempt to put it into practice.

When a child did something deemed valuable to society, he would be rewarded, and with enough repetition, it would become a part of the individual's learned behavior. One eminent behaviorist, John Watson, went so far as to say that if you gave him a dozen healthy infants, he could take any one at random and train it to become whatever he selected—doctor, lawyer, artist, merchant, even beggarman or thief, regardless of the talents, penchants, abilities, vocations and race of his ancestors.

Well, today we know it's not that simple. Man is a product of both genes *and* environment, which includes everything from food to the attitude of the care-giver who feeds him. An infant starts out with an incredibly complex genetic makeup and, through learning, modifies his behavior in response to a changing environment. We are still looking for answers to why we are the way we are, but the nature/nurture controversy has basically been stilled.

Although there will always be some who lean toward heredity and others who are inclined toward environment, we believe that we arrive at maturity through a synergistic relationship between the two. By his nature, man is born; by nurturing, so does he grow.

Society, beginning with parents, ending up with peers and the boss, molds a person's development—physical, mental and spiritual. The final product is to a large degree shaped in the early months and years of life, and although the body changes, basic temperament remains pretty much the same throughout a lifetime—although it might not be obvious to others.

Quite recently some scientists have questioned how much a child's early experiences and tendencies govern the type of adolescent and adult he will grow up to be. Their theory is that the early experiences may be permanently lost, and that what happens in the first year is not a harbinger of what's to come. While it may be true that we are not forever locked into repeating a bad experience and allowing it to govern our lives, we suspect that the early occurrences and their aftermath—whether we remember them or not—become ingrained, even though the trauma of a toddler may seem remote from present reality. However, it may be possible to compensate in some areas.

Studies of Korean orphans adopted into American homes indicate that although the children's start in life was troubled, six years later they were able to score as well as average American children on school achievement and IQ tests. But the success of a life cannot be measured by an intelligence test.

Consider yourself for a moment. If you were a shy, reticent child, the one who was terrified of starting kindergarten two months late because you had your appendix out on the first day of school, you may still feel that the rest of the world has the jump on you. You may be a success, you might have a fancy job with a big title, but there's always that insecurity, even if others aren't aware of it or can't see any reason why you—of all people—should feel that way. You may not always remember that first day of kindergarten when you apply for a new job, but in the middle of the night it creeps up on you. You know why you overcompensate with bravado. Or why you are still so shy.

Perhaps you were always the life of the party, started kindergarten with gusto and organized the kids during recess to play your games. You are probably still exhibiting those same outgoing leadership qualities, and may have a job in which you get to use your special social abilities.

Or going back before that, you may have been using big words in complete sentences before you were a year old. You most likely do not recall that your father proudly used to challenge neighbors and relatives to trip up his daughter with a big word. When you were older you were probably told about this again and again, and as you grew up you came to believe that indeed you did have a way with words.

If we seem to have deviated from eyes, and appear to be delving into the whole human experience, it is because it is impossible to separate the two. The growth and development of a human being is intimately linked with his vision, and it is impossible to study one without examining the other.

Today more than ever before we depend on our visual sense to get along in the world. Would your life be markedly altered if you woke up tomorrow and your sense of smell was gone? Would you have to quit your job and take special training to get along? Not unless your job was mixing perfumes. But if you lived in the forest and the vale, as our ancestors did, and hunted as a primary occupation, you would be severely hindered without a nose in good working order. Watch a dog when he's out hunting. His nose does twitch. A lot.

The late Dr. Arnold Gesell, whose observations of childhood led him to devote much research to vision, observed that a child's visual development compresses into a short time the countless stages of evolution which brought vision to its present advanced state in the human species. "The child's patterns of visual behavior go through progressive stages of maturity correlated with his changing postural control, his manual coordinations, his intelligence and even his personality."

It is widely thought today that certain physical attributes during fetal growth (such as the appearance of gills) and later patterns of behavior (such as creeping and crawling) are reminders of our heritage and reflect the evolutionary steps we have come through to reach our present upright form. The ultimate question is: what are we doing to ourselves today that will change the shape of man tomorrow?

The smell of danger and the sound of an animal coming toward Uncle Ramapithecus (who lived some 14 million years ago) made him jump for cover. Today the less aware we are of the roar of traffic and the smell of garbage, the better off we appear to be.

But even a slight tuning down of any of our senses—no matter which one—shuts off sensory information to the brain, that great computer which puts everything together and makes a decision about what is felt, heard, smelled, tasted or seen. That is how we learn about life, whether it be from running across a field on a pony or reading a book about riding a pony cross-country. The brain, like a computer, doesn't do anything without data. It simply uses the senses rather than punch cards.

The problem is that we have leftover eyes. They evolved through the eons to work well for the hunter and the countryman, but they aren't suited for the life we lead today. The urban academic uses his eyes in vastly different ways than did the man who hunted and gathered berries all day long. Today we rely on our eyes for between 80 and 90 percent of the information we receive about the world. Our eyes have always done their best to accommodate us, but they cannot change overnight—or in a century.

It is assumed that somewhere back in the evolutionary reaches, where the data is of necessity speculative, early forms of life had only one primitive eye. Later many creatures had eyes like fish—one on each side of the head. It is thought that in the twinkling of a few hundred million years eyes did the walking and slid forward to a place in front of the head where they could be used together. Long before man evolved, his ancestors developed 3-D vision. When other beneficial attributes came along, the anthropoid who became man took a giant step forward and put himself on top of the evolutionary heap all at once.

Now he could hunt the wild animals with better equipment: frontal vision, an upright walk, freely swinging hands which could be guided by eyes, a thumb to manipulate tools, language, imagination. He could devise tools and shoot a bow and arrow. To a greater or lesser degree, for better or for worse, man took charge of everyone and everything else. We have to assume it was for the best.

But in a relatively short time, a scant few million years later, we are asking our eyes to handle a job for which they were not really made. We learned how to write books; we put up cities and narrowed our visual perspective. When was the last time you gazed joyfully, peacefully, at a sunset going down over the mountains? We do not mean from the Rainbow Room on the 65th floor of the RCA building in Manhattan. That horizon with its up-and-down lines called buildings is not really restful to the eye.

The awake eye—at rest—is always gazing off into the horizon. That is why the peoples of the world tend to be what we call farsighted. But bring in literacy, and that farsightedness, the ability to see best afar, becomes a liability of sorts. What the world wants now are readers—folks who don't have any trouble focusing for long periods of time at nearpoint, say 16 inches away from the eye, which is where you are probably holding this book.

Our culture is losing sight of the fact that man is not simply an intellectual being, a refiner of abstract thought. Man also has arms and legs and feelings and genitals and skin which loves to be touched. We have motor skills which propel us through space, whether we crawl, walk or jog, and senses other than sight which should be enjoyed. But the way we are pursuing intellectualism above all else—except for the dropouts who said enough is enough—has us racing pell-mell toward the evolution of man into some kind of giant egghead, with sticks attached for arms and legs.

An infant is not yet caught in the twentieth-century intellectual trap, however, and when he starts out on his quest to learn about this world, he uses all that he is: touch, sight, smell, hearing and taste—and a brain. He opens up the cupboard and pulls out pots and pans to look at, to feel their cool hardness, to bang them on the floor and hear the clanking sound they make. Grownups may see pots only as receptacles; to a child a pot is a drum, a hat, a container for little toys, and yes, you can pour fluids in—and out—of it. To the youngster, the pot is as magnificent a tool as it probably was considered by the man or woman who invented the first one.

When we interfere with this integrating process in an individual we begin to run into trouble. There are millions of words on the book-shelves telling parents how to turn their children into Superbright Kids—the ones who do so well in IQ tests—but they concentrate solely on expanding the intellectual horizons and neglect or diminish the other aspects of what it is to be human. There are lots of times a child would be better off daydreaming or playing Red Rover than reading or work-ing a crossword puzzle for fun.

Far too many of us are growing up today with a highly developed intellect, but with our muscles and emotions arrested. Some of us haven't taken time to learn how good it feels to move and touch. We haven't bothered to experience our feelings, but immediately put them into words—and intellectualizing always involves making a judgement which separates us from the sensory flow of the moment.

Anthropologists generally consider ours a touch-deprived society. Aware that something is missing, we pay others to touch for us. Massage has long flourished where emotional and physical restraint is valued, in Japan and Sweden.

By thus limiting ourselves, we allow only one avenue to travel when it comes to dealing with different situations. Yet it is not always appropriate to talk our way out of—or into—a situation. Silence may be called for. Or reaching out and touching someone. In a crisis, the in-tellectual may only verbalize what is going on, rather than empathize with his own feelings or with others. He sits things out while bridges—and people—blow up around him. It's not really his fault; he simply hasn't learned how to act differently. He was too busy racking up IQ points to have time to learn how to feel.

In addition, we have moved from the warm climates ideally suited to man and have crowded ourselves into big cities all over the globe where the wind blows hot and cold. We have changed the way we live, but our bodies haven't kept pace. Reactions and equipment that were adequate for the Stone Age are often not good enough for the present. René Dubos notes: "Evolutionary fitness is always fitness for the past."

The price we are paying for changes we have wrought appears to be anxiety and disease that come in many forms—migraines to ulcers to heart attacks and all the other stops on the way—which were unknown in primitive cultures. If we have lost the ability to handle a difficult situation in any other way than verbalizing it, what do we do when that is inappropriate? Get a migraine so painful that we can't worry about the problem?

Rather than deal with the heart of the matter, society has developed a host of palliatives for treating the symptoms. Fortunately, new approaches are asking the body to help heal the mind, as therapy moves off the talking couch into the moving body. What Wilhelm Reich began in the late thirties with his concept of feelings locked into frozen muscles has been danced around a bit in the last few decades and mixed up with the ancient art of massage. Currently we have a veritable alphabet soup of body therapies from which to choose, and although they are all effective for one symptom or another, the assortment is bewildering to the person seeking relief. There is no ready answer as to what works best for a particular problem or personality. Help can come in many forms.

We can be Rolfed for body realignment, or lie through a Shaitsu massage for better circulation and a toned-up nervous system. The Reichians will jab us where it hurts to release the feelings stashed there, and zone therapists will work over our feet to coddle the nerve endings of our entire body. In the Feldencrais method, our limbs will be manipulated to increase awareness of our bodies so we may let them take over some of the jobs we have been intently and hopelessly delegating to will power alone. Dance therapists will get us moving to reveal our emotions, and at Esalen we will be fondled and touched until we can't help but learn how to give in and enjoy sensate pleasure apart from sex.

An approach to healing which integrates body, mind and environment—which is the norm rather than the novel in systems of medicine other than Western—may unlock a way to nurture the whole man, not just make him well when he is obviously ailing, but upgrade the level of what we consider health and well-being.

A healthy individual is one who knows how to operate with ease in all spheres of his being: muscle, mind, emotion. He is able to adapt to change, absorb a certain amount of stress and swing back into equilibrium quickly. It is not all that certain that if we cannot do this we will survive as a species.

"People feel that we are here by predestination and that because we are humans we will be able to survive even if we make mistakes," comments anthropologist Richard Leakey. "There have been thousands of living organisms of which a very high percentage have become extinct. There is nothing, at the moment, to suggest that we are not part of the same pattern."

However, our saving grace may be that ability which sets us apart from all other living things: the power to reflect on the past and plan for the future.

An Individual Life

Shallow men believe in luck and circumstance; strong men believe in cause and effect.
—Wisdom found in a fortune cookie

Now that we have looked at where we have come from and where we might be headed, let us examine what happens in an individual. Just as mankind takes a turn to the left or right when the environment dictates, so does an infant. We could assume that a child would progress along the normal lines of development—if there were no outside influences. But there's mom and pop and the rest of the world, and what happens in the interaction between child and environment, especially during the critical early months and years, is to a large extent what shapes the adult. The infant learns one task to be able to do another, each more complicated than the last, and this process continues, more or less, until we die.

Because our culture is so thoroughly modern while our bodies are not, it is crucial that we develop to the best of our abilities if we are to get along in the world. We've left visual development pretty much up to chance in the past. While that might have been good enough for the hunter-gatherers that our ancestors were, it will not do for the present where to be without good visual skills is to be limited by blinders. Aside from the obvious acuity difficulties rampant in a literate society, there are the unrecognized maladaptations—bad visual habits, as it were—which prevent us from reaching our potential and living life as fully and enjoyably as we might.

Right from the start a child's temperament will be evident. The folks who spend a lot of time watching infants say there are basically four personality types: easy, difficult, slow starter and highly active.

The easygoing infant is everybody's ideal. He's responsive to new stimuli but not overly excitable. Cries some, but not most of the time.

The difficult, irregular child is slow to adapt to change, finds plenty not to his liking and withdraws from new stimulation rather than joining in the fun. This one lets you know—loudly—when he doesn't like someone or something.

The slow starter doesn't like new things either, but isn't as vocal in his objection. He's resistant to change generally, but instead of wailing about it simply withdraws and lets the rest of the world go on about its confusing business. He needs frequent exposure without pressure to learn to accept a new stimulus or situation.

In contrast, the active type needs plenty of new toys and situations to keep him interested. He's bright and alert, and if he doesn't have enough to keep him interested he's likely to cause problems by creating his own novel situations—which is another way of saying he'll get into trouble. If this type of youngster doesn't have enough to keep him busy, his behavior is seen as misbehavior. He is likely to ignore your commands of *No!* And if they are repeated too often, he tunes out and withdraws.

Although heredity will have done its ineluctable typecasting at the moment of conception, we can modify the environment to suit the needs of each individual rather than exacerbate a troublesome tendency. If an infant is jumpy, don't make him more so by flicking on bright lights or jostling him around; what's called for are tender, soothing sounds and movements. Placid children can be stimulated somewhat more, but how much is possible remains a question. One study found, not surprisingly, that children who are hyperactive and do not sit still grow up to be people who by and large avoid intellectual pursuits, which require silence and reflection.

It takes about a dozen years for a pair of eyes to grow up and achieve adult vision and perception, even though the apparatus is largely organized and ready to go by the time the child is six. Practice with eyes starts well before birth, when they jerk around independently under sealed lids. At birth a child is able to move his eyes momentarily, but usually one at a time. He looks at you now with this eye, now with that. His focusing ability is within a few inches of his face. Eye movement is closely linked to body movement: when he looks, he stops moving, and when he moves, he stops looking. One thing at a time for now. He sees but does not yet understand. Vision is basically a reflexive response to light and size.

His optic nerves, which will ultimately transmit impulses to the brain, do not yet have their protective sheath of myelin and are not equipped to handle the electrical charges which result in vision. The newly born infant has a lot to get used to in the outside world, and right now the extra stimulation of seeing everything is more than he can handle. There's this whole other atmosphere to live and breathe in, you see.

Even in the first week the infant has some basic survival equipment built into his visual mechanism. He will try to avoid an object approaching his face; but if it is clear to him that the object will miss his face, he will watch it but not respond. The tests, incidentally, were done with a shadow to eliminate sound and wind; the visual cue was the only one to tell him that something was coming.

By the second week the child will start to make smiling facial movements, although he is not yet connecting that smile with happy feelings. This smile is thought to be a response like a kneejerk. It's just something to try out, along with sticking out his tongue, fluttering his eyes ever so charmingly, and opening and closing his mouth. He's got all the apparatus, and he's beginning to check out what he can do with it: eating, sucking, kissing, fondling, touching, moving and wetting his diaper are all new sensations to an infant. He must learn how they work.

He can't accomplish much, yet even in those early weeks he will be attracted to sounds and lights and will attempt to turn his eyes and head toward them. He will be quieted by touching and feeding and will demand them aplenty. In the womb there was the constant stimulation and warmth of the mother's body, and a newborn is hardly going to get used to his new world in a few days or weeks.

Some hospitals allow the mother to spend time each day in the nursery when a child is in an incubator, and even though a plastic box separates them, the infant is able to have someone to watch, a face which will become recognizable as mom. While the senses of touch and smell are cut off, what is being acknowledged is that it is essential for the infant to form an attachment to another human being right from the start.

A number of studies with animals—monkeys, puppies and goats— show that the development of a crucial connection to a moving object is possible only during short periods in the early life of the infant. A baby goose has only a few hours in the first days of life in which to learn to follow his mother. Animals raised with mothers, who do all the motherly things such as cleaning and feeding and otherwise random nuzzling, learn quickly and pass these traits on to their young. Monkeys raised without mothering turn out to be "hopeless, helpless and heartless," in the words of two researchers.

Harry and Margaret Harlow at the University of Wisconsin found that monkeys don't form attachments to a mother because she is the source of food, but because she is soft and pliant and feels good to cling to. They discovered this by raising an infant monkey in isolation and giving him a choice of two surrogate mothers: one made of hard wire mesh, the other a form covered by terry cloth. The terry cloth mom was always chosen—even though the wire one offered food, too. When the terry cloth mom was removed, the monkeys threw themselves on the floor of the cage and screamed in terror. If we learn anything from this, it is not to be stingy with touch.

Eckhard Hess at the University of Chicago found that this *imprinting* to another of the species (at least in ducks) is deepest and firmest if it occurs between 13 and 16 hours after hatching, which is when a duckling starts following his mother around. If this is delayed beyond a day, it collides with another critical period of innate behavior—fear of moving objects, which occurs by the middle of the second day. Clearly, if the duckling does not have the opportunity to make the required responses in the right order at the right time, it doesn't have much of a chance in the wild. Although recent research indicates that this behavior can be somewhat altered, animals normally attach themselves to the first moving thing they see—whether that be another animal of the same species, the researcher or a wooden decoy. One student of Hess was able to imprint a duckling to herself and a quail to the duckling by being the only moving object there during the critical period. They followed her everywhere they could.

Now, obviously, we're not ducks or monkeys, but the message should be clear: Certain types of learning must occur within specified time limits, and if this maturing process is obstructed, the pattern may never be established, and what is to follow does not have a firm grounding.

Although it would be out of the question to use human babies to study behavior in such a coldly clinical situation, it has been tried in the past. Back in the thirteenth century, Emperor Frederick II wondered what language children would speak if they heard no one talk at all. Would they speak in their parents' tongue? Invent a language?

He got a group of boy babies together and told their nurses to care for their physical needs but otherwise to pay no attention to them. Above all, they were not to be spoken to. The emperor never found out what language the children might use to communicate, because they all died.

Although the term *imprinting* is usually replaced by the word *bonding* in reference to humans, it is recognized that infants must form an attachment to a particular adult during their early months if they are to develop normally. One psychologist suggests that the infant's first social smile (at four to six weeks) is equivalent to the "following" response in ducks. Sound and motion are the critical stimuli in ducklings; for babies, one particular part of the human face—the eyes—is thought to be the first moving object seen. Tiny babies can't absorb large objects, and of all the features on a face, the eyes are the most mobile. Not only do they move around, they sparkle and shine.

The mother's tendency to cuddle a baby and give him the opportunity to see and touch, just as animals care for their young in the normal order of things, is thought to be built into the genes. A baby, usually held and cuddled a lot, learns right from the beginning what a human being is like and what is expected of him: to give and to receive love. The mother's attitude to the child and to life in general is part of the picture the child learns. If, for example, she is fearful, she undoubtedly passes this cue on to the child in subtle ways.

His focusing ability—limited though it is—gives him a way to recognize mom, the one with whom he feels safe, the one who nurtures him with food and picks him up when he cries. But if these things don't happen—if he is ignored when he wants and needs love and attention—he is bound to grow up without a clear idea of his own identity and importance.

Not being able to see the love in a mother's eyes is thought to be a major reason why people blind from birth often have difficulty with interpersonal relationships at any age. Orphans who are denied close contact with a mother in those first few months after birth also have a hard time in establishing trustful, loving relationships with others, and this pattern seems to haunt many of them all their lives. In addition, children institutionalized early are found to be retarded in their intellectual and emotional development. They have lower-than-normal IQs, are behind in language skills and tend to be apathetic, unambitious and relatively unresponsive to approval.

We do know, of course, that behavior can be modified. While early experiences do not necessarily dictate the kind of adult you will grow up to be, the degree to which modifying behavior is possible, particularly in feelings, is questionable. We may learn how to compensate for early emotional trauma, but we never entirely lose its effects. The teenager who is rejected by her father may have a difficult time later forming a close relationship with a man. Always on guard against being rejected again, she may maintain a distance and be ready to walk out, rather than opening herself up to the possibility of hurt—and love.

At six months, children raised in institutions are found to lack a clear idea of their identity; the high level of frustration they experience in trying to get their needs taken care of greatly reduces their ability to attend to what is going on around them.

Animal studies show that rats that are deprived of something basic, such as water, have a much harder time learning how to get through a maze than rats that aren't hungry or thirsty. Chimps react the same way, with the best performance in learning a task (with food as the reward) occurring when there is moderate motivation, not an extreme at either end. A chimp that hasn't just had dinner—or is ravenous—is likely to achieve the best. When the obvious needs are taken care of, learning occurs more swiftly, just as an adult cannot attend to business if an emotional problem is chipping away at his consciousness. Perhaps this explains why the greatest advances of man occur in the temperate zones, where the weather makes food not as available as cocoanuts and bananas in the tropics, nor as inaccessible as fish and game among the ice floes.

Some consider autism, a condition in which a child withdraws to the extent where there is little or no communication, a response to an environment which is seen only as hostile and destructive. Others, however, consider the malady largely biochemical. It is probably both, but we do not know which factor turns the switch on. Once it gets going, it may be that one reaction triggers the other.

As the animal studies indicate, moderation is the key to the most efficient learning. The same is true with human infants. Babies who were overwhelmed with geegaws and gimcracks hanging over their cribs and lay on gaudily patterned sheets were found to lag behind in developing eye/hand coordination. The group that had a moderate amount of things to look at were ahead. Their sheets were plain, and interesting objects were attached to the sides of the crib, so that they could look at them *when they wanted to*. It appears that the babies who were overstimulated simply tuned out. They also cried more than the other group.

Although the infant sounds as if he were computing the incoming data at a high level of sophistication, he is hardly aware of what is going on. To begin with, he is getting used to the idea that there is a difference between "me" and "you"—it's usually mom, but it can be any primary care-giver. There is very little a new baby sees that he understands, but he does perceive differences.

When five-day-old infants were given a choice of things to look at —a face, a bull's eye, a section of newsprint, a plain white circle, a fluorescent yellow circle or a red circle, the object which held the most attention was the face. None of the 18 infants in the survey chose to look at the plain colors for very long.

The same investigator, Robert Fantz, also showed that young babies can discriminate among quite similar patterns. Infants less than two weeks old were cradled in a special chamber, and pictures were shown from above. When the infant was looking at the picture, the image was reflected in the cornea, and the length of time the picture caught the baby's eye was recorded. Five different arrangements of black and white squares were shown; some were in up-and-down lines, others in checkerboard patterns, and others randomly drawn on the paper. Almost half the babies showed the most interest in the pattern in which the squares were neatly lined up in a horizontal arrangement.

The choice itself is interesting, because the infants picked the design that the human eye at this stage of evolution is best suited for: gazing at the horizon.

By the fifth or sixth week the infant has gained some control of his head and can hold it erect, although it will bob around a bit. His eyes will follow a moving person across a room, and he pays more and more attention to light rather than sound. His eye control is on its way, but his hands are still locked into fists. He is learning how to control his environment slowly but steadily, and always with his eyes before his limbs. Even at this early stage the visual sense is taking dominance. Acuity has doubled from what it was at the beginning, meaning that within three feet, the radius of the area to which he now relates, he will attend to an object half the size of what caught his eye the previous month. Now he looks at an object under four inches in diameter, although he is still unable to adjust his focusing to see clearly.

When his eyes are examined with a retinoscope, there is an occasional brightening and darkening of the focusing reflex, almost as if he is shutting out one eye and turning on the other alternately. Examined earlier, it appeared that one eye at a time will be on, and then both off. Now it's one or the other.

As soon as the little tyke can open his fist to grab, he starts doing so and putting everything he can into his mouth. Mom might think the habit is unsanitary, but look at it from his point of view: Everything is new to him, and most of his pleasurable activity is with his mouth: a nipple which nourishes him. Why shouldn't everything else be tried out the same way? It might taste good.

What he is doing occurs in this sequence: see, grab, eat. One could view this as a basic survival instinct which teaches him eye/hand coordination. Someday it will help him learn how to hold a spoon or open his mail. At the same time he is learning about the sizes and shapes of different objects. There's an awfully big world out there, with a lot of different things in it. That baby has to learn how to put them into categories, make some conceptual judgement about them and understand that what appears to be true one day may seem different the next. The process never quite ends.

At approximately 10 weeks, alpha waves, a type of electrical activity of the brain, begin. Alpha normally occurs when our eyes are closed, but prior to 10 weeks it seems that the infant is not able to discriminate visual from non-visual information, and so no alpha is recorded. There may be no difference in the infant's cortex between sight and non-sight. The infant isn't ready to handle the heady experience of *really* seeing as he will later on.

Between 10 and 12 weeks, the optic nerves become completely covered with their layer of myelin, which acts much like insulation around electrical wire. The signals sent from a young infant's brand-new eyes to its brand-new brain are actually carried by a group of nerves that are still developing. The brain is plugged in, but the wires don't work.

When we see, light becomes electrical energy of a sort, travels along the visual pathways and ends up in the back of the cortex, where it is interpreted. Until myelination is completed, it appears that vision is controlled by the old brain, or spinal cord and medulla, which operate the basic reflex systems such as breathing and pupillary reflex. This is the entire brain in some lower animals: the primitive brain gets the primitive signal.

This recent observation is based on research at Temple University which shows that at the time myelination occurs, a definite change in vision can be observed. When 16 infants under two months were shown black and white circles or horizontal lines, the only preferences noted were for size: the bigger the better. However, at two months, all the infants showed a definite preference for circles, regardless of size. Investigators Diana Woodruff and Kathleen Gerrity propose that this visual shift indicates the time when vision moves from the old brain to the new brain, which by now has developed to the point where it is functional.

Vision has become less a simple response to light and is steadily more interpretive. An infant is becoming capable of selecting what he wants to look at. A functioning cortex also processes other information for the child, and the beginning of memory is soon observed, for the youngster shows some recognition of specific faces and shapes in his environment. He begins to discriminate, which means he will be more interested in a new rattle than in that same old shaker—even if it is silver and came from Tiffany's.

The eyes are beginning to learn how it feels to work together, and will converge on mom or pop as they come toward him. Before that, one eye was looking, one eye tuning out. As the eyes begin to function as a unit, during the third month, he is now able to get his hands into the act since they have gained enough strength to reach out and knock over a toy. Great fun. For Junior. Now he's able to track an object past the middle of his body; before that, an object could be followed from the side to the center, but not beyond. The other eye would have to take over. And at this time the child's control of his head lets him turn it to watch.

Using both eyes together gives him more accurate depth perception. To see objects in space, not just a flat picture, one needs to have the use of both eyes. The baby will show a definite preference for a real face—especially one that's familiar—and will also respond readily to a sculpted head or a mask, but less quickly to a drawing.

Interestingly enough, two researchers found that a baby from three to approximately six months will usually smile at any face that looks human—even if it's a frightening mask from a Japanese No drama or a Greek tragedy. The child doesn't yet know what's a scary expression, and all the faces represent only one thing: another of his kind. He smiles his *hello* back in recognition. However, that smile can be shut off like a light if the face turns sideways. A profile does not yet give the child enough information.

Others report that by the fourth or fifth month a child may "freeze" when a strange adult comes near, sitting completely still, scarcely moving a muscle, barely breathing. In animals this response is taken as an index of fear. But this reaction is mild compared to the anxiety of being separated from mom and the fear of strangers that begins at about eight months and lasts well into the second year. But when a bond has been made with another member of the human race, the infant is ready to start peeking at what is going on beyond that single care-giver.

With mom as a stable home base, he starts wandering around more. As long as he can hear mom in the kitchen, he feels safe enough to investigate a different room in the house. Knowing mom is nearby gives him the confidence to look past her and begin to learn what else is out there.

When the first social smile occurs, a human voice or a touch will elicit the smile better than any other cue, including visual. Blind babies at this stage smile just as much as do the sighted, but this drops off later.

Somewhere in the middle of the third month the infant is beginning to be able to remember what he's seen and to predict what is going to happen. If someone walks behind a screen or a door, the infant understands the person did not vanish altogether, and will turn his head and eyes to look at the point where the person is expected to come out. Yet if you put a toy under a blanket, he does not yet understand that it is under the blanket. He acts as if it has disappeared, and to his mind, it has. But the ability to predict events, such as mother walking behind a screen, will eventually help him understand that things do not disappear just because he can't see them.

The fourth month is basically a time of linking eye and hand. This will give the child the feeling that he can manipulate space to his liking, preparing him for the time when he will move out into that space, crawling away from mom, somewhere around the eighth month. Then he identifies and depends on one—sometimes two—people to be there when he needs and wants them. Strangers won't do.

By the fifth month he can roll over and raise his chest, and is beginning to try to sit up by himself. Body movements are guided by the brain, and the body has developed to the point where it can carry out simple commands. The brain directs: Raise chest. Grab that rag doll and throw it on the floor. It's his way of understanding what happens in the real world, getting him ready for his own movements through space.

Language may start at this time, with the child saying a simple word or two: *mama, dada.* Mama and dada get as much joy out of that as Junior.

Before his sixth month the infant clearly recognizes that he has one mother and only one. If the child is presented with three mirrored images of mom at the same time, he will protest, and loudly. Before that, he hardly reacts, or is delighted and will interact with all three mothers in turn. Now that he knows that he has only one mom, he protests vigorously when he is separated from her. Prior to this time, the baby acts as if he believes that when one mother leaves another will automatically pop up somewhere. But now, if a child wakes up and finds the baby-sitter there instead of mom, he is not going to like it one bit and will let her know, usually with vigor. The more she tries to comfort him, the more upset he seems to get. It's extremely frustrating for the adult trying to assure the child that everything is all right.

The primary care-giver to whom the child clings does not have to be the mother. Some babies do not care so much about separation from mother, but protest when father leaves. Grandparents can likewise be the object of a child's affection. Although it is thought that at the beginning the child forms an attachment to just one person, one extensive study found that by the time separation anxiety sets in fully a third of the babies protested being separated from two people.

The study, done in the mid-sixties, also found that approximately 20 percent of the babies were attached to a person who had no part in their physical care whatsoever, a fact which should make mothers who work rest peacefully. The obvious suggestion is that it is not the amount of time that a care-giver spends with a child, but the quality of the interaction that matters.

In the sixth month an infant is ready to go. He is fairly competent at using both eyes together. Eye/hand coordination should be quite well developed, so that when Junior reaches out to knock toys, bottles, clothespins—anything—off his high-chair tray, he succeeds. Creeping usually begins at the eighth month, and he may begin to walk (holding on) at 12 months, walk alone at 15 months and run stiffly at 18 months.

When he begins to walk he will not want to go far from the home base. He knows where mom is, and he wants to make sure that she stays put while he ventures out into the great unknown. He may continue this pattern to some degree for the rest of his life. Later, he'll go to school—and come home at the end of the day; later still, he'll go away to college, and return for the summer, and after that he might move out of town but will return home regularly to visit.

Between 18 months and two years, he will develop his language skills to communicate with the outside world, and by the middle of his second year he should have acquired a strong enough sense of himself to allow him to move farther and farther away from home.

By three he's gone. He'll visit the kid next door or down the block. He's even able to stay overnight and finds it a great adventure. He knows that home will be there when he returns.

From two-and-a-half on, vision and language integrate to develop his ability to categorize objects and events in his life, laying the groundwork for adult intelligence.

The developmental road map we've laid out here sounds regular and predictable—and it is, within some degree of flexibility. Individual differences should always be taken into account. One child will be doing something ahead of the norm, another will be lagging behind in a skill.

But all of the abilities should be attained within a few months of what is expected, and these include the entire gamut of what it is to be human: motor skills, movement of the entire body, visual ability, perception and language. Out of these aptitudes interpersonal relationships and intelligence will grow, based on what nature put there and the type of nurturing received from the environment.

While the basic progression appears to be unlearned because it is so predictable, that is not quite the case. The developmental steps are programmed to occur at certain times, provided they have had proper stimulation. Lacking that, they fail to take place appropriately.

Consider the institutionalized children we mentioned earlier. One researcher, who originally thought that if a child's physical well-being was taken care of he would develop normally, ultimately changed his mind after he had visited orphanages in Iran. Wayne Dennis had based his earlier perception on the fact that he and his wife had tried to raise their twin girls with almost no social interaction; they simply saw to it that the girls' physical needs were taken care of. By the ninth month, scientific detachment broke down, and they gave up trying to raise their daughters in an unnatural environment with little outside stimulation from them. Until that point, the children had progressed normally. They turned over, smiled, sat up and babbled like any other child. From this Dennis assumed that development is genetically determined.

However, when he visited the orphanages, Dennis found that while most American babies are sitting up by nine months, fewer than half of the Iranian infants were able to do so—even at 21 months. And when it came to walking, the Iranian children were also well behind, many by as much as a year. In two of the institutions the children were only removed from their cribs every other day, when they were bathed. They lay on their backs until they could sit up by themselves, and then they were often plunked down in rows, with no toys and virtually no individual attention from the attendants.

Yet in another institution, where an attendant had only three or four children to care for, they were held when fed, had toys and received much more personal attention. These children were only slightly behind the norm.

Our norm, that is. But what would happen in a culture where the mothers are totally child-centered? Where the infant receives fondling and encouragement every step of the way? They develop much faster than our children.

A study in the late 1950s of more than 300 infants in Uganda, where ancient custom dictates that the child receives attention we would consider excessive, the children were sitting up at seven weeks, in contrast to the western norm of 18 weeks. At seven months the Ugandan infant was walking to a box and taking toys out of it. Our infants usually walk between 12 and 15 months. Some research attributes superior adult coordination to early physiological maturing of the Africans. This seems to be the case on the whole, but the babies from Uganda were also ahead of ours in adapting to new situations, social relationships and language skills.

How were the babies treated? Their mothers were with them day and night. The Ugandan infant is talked to, stroked, fed whenever hungry. He is watched intently for cues as to what he wants to do. If an infant appears to be struggling to sit up, his mother helps him. Her life revolves totally around the child.

Most of the infants in the fast-developing group were from the lower classes of Uganda. A few were from a higher class, which is to say they were more westernized in their approach to child-rearing. Feedings were done on schedule, there was less physical contact with the mother and more attention to rigid training. And these children were not nearly as precocious as the babies reared in the traditional manner of the Ugandans.

It may be that in the right-to-work doctrine inherent in today's feminism we are granting women a certain kind of self-fulfillment, but at a cost to the generations to come. The data would indicate that perhaps a mother's—or father's—place is in the home, especially in the infant's first year. Considering the current population projections, the course to take may be the age-old one which has been the source of much discontent: choosing either a career or children. It is hard to concentrate on a board meeting or a deadline when something in a woman tells her she would rather be at home playing with baby. Is it unlikely that her genes are calling her home?

There are a number of studies which feminists love to hate (and which of late have been largely ignored), but one visual finding makes the point: When women look at pictures of babies, regardless of an overall deadpan demeanor, their pupils expand, as if in delight. Just the way a man's pupils dilate when he looks at a picture of a pretty girl. The way of the world—of generations through the eons that have brought us to this point—cannot be dismissed by an act of will.

We are not suggesting that women leave their jobs behind and return to the hearth. Or that they be given less pay for equal work because their heart's not in it. We are saying that the twentieth-century woman still must consider her priorities. If she opts to have both children and a career, she should at least consider that maybe taking a year or two off would make her—and baby—happier in the long run.

But as things stand now, if a woman chooses to leave a good job to raise her baby, she is subjected to a barrage of criticism from friends and acquaintances who work outside the home. By not allowing a woman to make such a personal choice without criticism we are impinging on her freedom and going against the grain of civilization.

Of course, as far as the baby is concerned, it need not be the mother who is the primary care-giver. The father could give the primary nurturing. It doesn't seem to matter who does the rearing, just that it be done.

Some of the newer studies implicitly say, *so what?* to the fact that infants reared with lots of love and affection seem to have an easier time growing up, and that their rate of growth is faster than that of other babies. Such support of an infant does not change the order of learned behavior, but if each stage has an adequate foundation, the next becomes easier to acquire. If the early stages are stable, they provide a broader base from which others flow. And in the twentieth century, because we have moved into cities all over the globe and drastically altered our environment—as no other species has ever done—it is necessary to develop and sharpen our abilities, not leave them to chance the way we did in the wild.

Although information on babies reared in inhospitable homes is difficult to come by due to the number of variables and the fact that a researcher cannot actually move in, a study reported by Murial Beadle in her excellent book, *A Child's Mind,* is revealing. Joyce Robertson of the Hampstead Child Guidance Clinic in London was able to observe a group of children and their mothers over a period of years, since the center is both a clinic and a nursery.

She began her observation when she noted that there were gross differences of muscular and motor development among some children at the nursery. When she went back to her early records, she discovered that the "clumsy ones were those whose mothering during the first year had been regarded as unsatisfactory." She began studying motor coordination and went on to look at the entire personality, since the two appear irretrievably linked. Her conclusion:

> *A baby mothered without warmth will develop broadly on the same lines as other babies. He will focus his eyes, smile, babble, find his limbs; but he will do it largely alone. There will be no*

fusion between the baby's achievement and the mother's pleasure and support; and for lack of his mother as an intermediary there will be less reaching out to the environment. The balance between adequate stimulation from his surroundings and potentially over-whelming experiences will not be maintained, and the baby may try to take over part of his own protection.

As early as eight to 10 weeks of age, the consequences are low quality and quantity of body movement, slow responses, serious facial expression, and eyes that are incongruously alert and watchful. The mother will say, "But he is so contented," mean-ing that he is undemanding or, "He is happiest when alone," un-aware that he may be withdrawing. With the passage of time these deficiencies become more gross. The uncomforted baby who swal-lows his tears at seven months may not cry at 12 months.

A baby will adjust to almost any condition and survive—but at a cost.

And a pair of eyes will adjust to almost any condition and sur-vive—but at a cost. Consider that approximately 100 million are in glasses, and add that to the high percentage of us who have other, *mostly undiscovered* visual difficulties which reflect themselves not only in our eyes but in our personalities, and which somehow limit us from operating as the free agents we should be.

How critical unhindered visual development is can be understood if we look at some animal studies where the process was arrested. If a monkey was made unable to open his eyes at birth but later allowed to, he was never able to develop fully useful vision. It appears that when the eyes are closed, and thus unable to receive the stimulation of light, the cells in the brain responsible for image-making atrophy and die. Light is a nutrient for vision just as milk is for growth, hearing and speech are nutrients for language, and problem-solving is a nutrient for intelligence.

When monkeys were allowed to see light—as if through an opaque window—but not images in focus, or the patterned light of pictures and shapes and colors, they also did not develop full vision. Their perceptual abilities suffered, and they were not able to discriminate what was being seen.

The same was true when the experiment was conducted on one eye only. If one eye was blocked and one wasn't, only the free eye learned how to see and was never able to teach the other eye what it had learned. There was no crossover. They had developed amblyopia.

What we can glean from these studies is that eyes must have both light and pattern to grow right. Mother's face. The blue rattle. The silver cup. The infant needs these things to learn how to see and to relate to this new and strange world around him.

Other research stresses the importance of the eye/body coordination. Kittens that were not allowed to move freely, nor see where they were going, were not able to get their eyes and paws coordinated later, or figure out where things were in space.

Kittens were raised in pairs. One was carried everywhere in a special gondola, the other was allowed to roam freely. When one kitten walked, the other was carried—but he saw everything the other kitten did. Later on the one that had been carried was set free. His eye/body coordination was off, his depth perception poor.

Kittens that had freedom but couldn't see their paws due to a special collar worn about the neck also had difficulty in learning how to get around, for they were not able to guide their movements. For instance, they couldn't figure out how to reach for a ball of yarn. Their paws just plunked down anywhere. Babies are not kittens, but we can infer from this research that any disruption of the normal process of maturation, specifically with the environmental ingredients of light, pattern and the ability to see what you are doing, obstructs growth and development of vision and coordination of what is seen with what the body does.

Although we do not restrict the movement of children for the sake of research, we can look at what happens when culture does it.

Children who are swaddled have been found to be behind in their motor development. The gypsy children of Albania were wrapped up and attached to a board left in one place most of the day. When examined at 12 months, they were far below our standards for eye/hand coordination. Children likewise swaddled but who got around on the back of their mother, as is the practice of American Indians, also had less coordination, but not nearly to such a degree.

Hopi Indians, who practice swaddling, show a great deal of astigmatism, which we consider may be the result of eyes trying to make up for poor posture and restricted movement.

Other research indicates that not only do eyes need light and pattern, they also must be stimulated with the variety of images that exist in the world: straight lines, both vertical and horizontal, circles and squares. If denied access to a certain visual shape during a particularly sensitive phase of development—when the gates are open, in a sense—laboratory animals were never able to regain mastery of that particular shape. Kittens raised so that they see only horizontal lines grow up to be animals who walk into the legs of chairs. They do not perceive the vertical plane of the legs of the chair.

And as we mentioned earlier, people who grow up without all shapes in their environment are never able to understand those that are not a part of the culture. Zulus, whose environment is comprised of wavy lines and circles, are never able to make sense of straight lines. They cannot, for instance, understand a photograph of an object whose edges are vertical and horizontal.

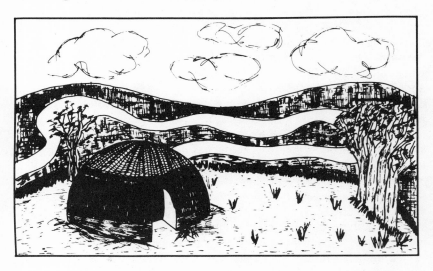

The Zulus live in an environment dominated by circular shapes.

The reason for this is that the *feature detectors* of the brain, an apparatus that discerns the difference between one shape and another, never developed because they were not properly stimulated according to schedule. The equipment was there, but deprived of the necessary nourishment, it atrophied.

Our culture modifies our particular system to meet our needs. City folk, used to looking at the up-and-down lines of buildings, tend to emphasize such sharp contours.

There is a story about a Russian farmer from the Ukraine who went to Moscow one day and ended up at the movies. His amazement bespoke his enjoyment, but asked later what the story was about, he had no idea. He was overwhelmed with this new sensory experience but was unable to make sense out of what he was seeing. He could only receive the signals; he could not interpret them. In a sense, his reaction was like a young infant's, who receives visual signals but cannot make sense of them.

Or consider the city slicker who goes hunting. In the eyes of the aborigines who make their daily living this way, he is seriously backward. He looks out at the plain, but does not see the animal in the distance—even though he may look at the same hill, the same clump of trees. He cannot interpret that fine dot as wild game. He looks, but he does not perceive. Coin collectors and others with hobbies that demand selective seeing also develop visual skills the rest of us do not have.

But perhaps the most graphic illustration of what can happen when our visual system is denied proper stimulation occurs with babies and adults who are blind from birth due to cataracts. In the beginning, babies seem to proceed almost normally. They smile at the sound of a human voice, they kick their legs like other babies. But if they are denied access to light and pattern, those nutrients necessary for healthy vision, for too long a time, it becomes nearly impossible for them ever to develop normal vision even after the cataracts are removed.

Babies born with cataracts should have them removed early.* Otherwise, the lack of sight produces permanent alterations in the structure of the brain, and they are never able to develop fully useful vision. The baby who has cataracts removed too late, even though his eyes can receive clear images, does not know what to do with them.

If vision is lost after six months, however, the adverse reaction to the child's development is less acute, but the effects can still be severe, up to the age of two-and-a-half.

Although we do not know exactly what happens in the case of humans, animal research indicates that those areas of the brain initially reserved for one visual skill can be taken over by another. If one good eye operates it takes over those sections of the brain usually reserved for the other. These effects, whether they are noted in monkeys, cats or frogs, occur only early in development.

How severely blindness affects the understanding of spatial concepts—or the relationship of one idea to another—depends on the age at which blindness occurred. Early is always worse. One study showed

---

* Recent animal research has shown that some cataracts—even advanced cases—can be reversed with a new drug which has been developed to replace cortisone.

that a group of congenitally blind children could pass a university entrance examination in Euclidean geometry, but their memorization of the theorems did not include even a basic understanding of how they work. They could not solve a single problem based on geometric principles involving the spatial relationships of a three-dimensional world.

There are about 60 cases on record of adults who were blind from birth but later—usually because of the removal of cataracts—were able to join the world of the sighted. Those who were highly educated while blind were able to adapt to their strange new environment, but not all. Some had severe emotional problems when they became sighted individuals which they could not overcome. Others simply shut their eyes to return to a life of darkness.

Such was the case of a woman in her mid-thirties who was a competent switchboard operator at an institute for the handicapped. She had been blind from birth, with defective corneas, but a transplant operation gave her sight. She was thrilled with what seemed like a miracle.

Incredibly, she soon found she couldn't even handle her old job—the one she could do effortlessly blind. Now that she could see, she could not integrate what her eyes could see with what her hands could do. The harder she tried, the more confused and frustrated she became. She was able to do the job when she closed her eyes—and that ultimately became her solution. Months later she wished that she could return to the world of the sightless. She shut her eyes and acted as if she were blind.

Because timing appears to matter so much, it is crucial that children who are developing a visual problem be put on the right track before it takes them into difficulties which seem far removed from poor sight. An emotional tendency may lead to a visual malfunction, which aggravates the emotional problem, and the dominoes start to fall. Visual difficulties do not go away by themselves—even if you can't see the problem.

Frequently, for example, a crossed eye that "straightens" by itself or with surgery simply shuts off. There's nothing wrong with the workings of the eye; the brain was just getting confused by the images the eye was sending and so turned off the mechanism by which it received data from that eye. You don't know it, and the child doesn't know it, because he's got one good eye doing all the work. When the turned-off eye is called upon to function by itself, such as during an examination for acuity, it will work, but usually to a lessened degree.

One little boy whose turned eye had appeared to straighten was examined at four-and-a-half. It was found that while the eye had "outgrown" the inward turn, the brain was shutting off vision from that eye. However, a permanent change due to lack of use had not yet occurred. Acuity measured 20/80 in that eye.

He was given a patch to wear on his "blind" eye so that it wouldn't have to suppress vision *not* to see—even if it tried it couldn't. He wore the patch at home but balked at wearing it to nursery school or while playing with friends. He picked out a pair of glasses, and the lens over the troubled eye was stippled with clear nail polish, thereby obstructing vision almost as well as the patch.

After three weeks the eye measured 20/40. The patch was then changed to the better eye. Focus activities were added for a few weeks. He would play cards with his mother. Each would have the same cards in front of them. When mom picked one up he would have to find the same card before she counted to five. Smaller and smaller cards were used to force him to be more and more precise. Some eye/hand coordination procedures were also done.

Some months later, he was given glasses with lenses that were half green and half red. A special red/green/clear filter was constructed to be attached to the television set. Since the red in his lenses would neutralize the green on the screen, and the green in the lenses neutralize the red, he had to use both eyes to get a total picture through the filters. As soon as he blocked his vision, a portion of the screen would fade into a blanket of gray. He started out sitting two feet from the set, because at that distance he was barely blocking vision; beyond that he was. At first he reported that the screen had black spots that would come and go, but to see *all* of his favorite programs his brain started making the adjustment not to turn off. It was visual biofeedback at work. In time the black spots at two feet went away, and he moved to three feet and so on, until they didn't appear at any distance. At the end of three months both eyes were working together.

And yet to look at him before, you wouldn't have suspected anything was the matter. After all, his eye had straightened by itself.

An individual goes through so many and varied psychological and physiological stages that they can be compared to the coming and going of ocean tides.

Birth is expansion. Within a week a child fits everything together; by four weeks, he smoothly coordinates what he has already learned. Between eight and twelve weeks is the break-up state; what once went well doesn't seem to work as smoothly during this period. A temporary quiet follows between sixteen to twenty weeks, when a child sorts out what has gone wrong. After this, a period of intense inwardizing—perhaps a sort of reflection—takes place; we see it as a time of outward stability and order during which a child makes logical sense of all that he has learned. Then the process is repeated over again, and a second period of expansion occurs between 24 and 28 weeks. Later on, the length of the stages vary, but this process of predictable change seems to go on through our lifetime.

As individuals we have our own emotional and physical crises—a marriage breaks up, a new one forms, a job is lost, another is gained—but as a group these fit into a predictable pattern, and one crisis must be resolved at a specific time so that another can occur a decade later.

A thirty-five-year-old woman, for instance, finds herself questioning whatever life it is she has chosen: if she is mothering a brood, she wonders what else she might have done and whether it's too late to try it. A childless woman with her name on a business card and the key to the executive washroom wonders if she can still find a mate and possibly fulfill the urge to procreate.

Life has a rhythm which has been defined and refined over the centuries to allow for our survival in a multitude of climates and a variety of lifestyles. Naturally, the goal is to insure that the race continues and creatively adapts to the environment we are shaping for ourselves; but the species should not pay too high a price. The way the world is going as we ascribe a higher and higher premium to intellectualism is changing us. True, many of us have our basic needs for food and shelter taken care of, and we are able to do that with a minimum of physical labor. But our back aches and our eyes are weak. We know it doesn't feel right. We get sick with diseases previously unknown. We wonder what's wrong and seek out a psychiatrist. We cry ourselves to sleep at night, whether or not the tears flow.

But, consider this: because we can think, we have the ability to question our direction.

Wilhelm Reich, along these same lines, suggested that life more or less follows an orgasmic pattern. There is the climb to the peak, the release of the orgasm, the receding flow before the next high point. The I Ching or *Book of Changes,* based on Chinese wisdom from the century before Confucius, celebrates the same pattern of life; a time of high excitement preceded and followed by a time of relaxation and calm. Life is a heartbeat, an ocean tide, the cycle of the moon.

6
Vitamins and Vision

Externally, all is well, one has meat and drink. But one is
exhausted by the commonplaces of life, and there seems to be
no way of escape. Then help comes from a high place.

Except for nibbling on a carrot now and then—which was supposed to have something to do with seeing at night—no one in the
past related nutrition to vision. But our eyes, like any other part of
our body, are affected by the environment, in this case food. And in
the same way that light and pattern are nutrients for sight, vitamins
and minerals are nutrients for our bodies, eyes included.

Although research demonstrating the importance of vitamins and
minerals has been available for many years, it has not been widely
circulated or heeded; those who preached the message of nutrition
were thought to be alarmists or food faddists. Except for the general
belief that one should eat a balanced meal, traditional medicine has
for years relegated nutrition to a back seat as far as health is concerned. The American Medical Association pays scant heed to nutrition. Of 122 medical schools in the country, only a dozen or so have
defined nutrition programs, with courses that include more than the
basics of good eating habits.

Lately, however, there is a growing awareness that vitamins and
minerals play a crucial role in our well-being, and that the general level
of health of almost everyone can be upgraded by supplementing diet
with vitamins and minerals. At the same time, doctors have become
more interested in nutrition and vitamin and mineral supplements as
biochemists began to report surprising results, coinciding with the message of the organic food and vitamin advocates.

There exists a debate today whether one should take supplements,
or attempt to obtain vitamins and minerals in enough quantity in food.

135

The discoveries of the last decade suggest amounts that are nearly impossible to take in simply through food. For instance, the suggested dosage of Vitamin C is one to five grams daily. An orange, a common natural source of Vitamin C, contains approximately 60 milligrams of C; thus you would have to eat 17 oranges a day to get even a single gram.

Also, much of the food available today at the supermarket or take-out counter has a good portion of the vitamins and minerals processed out of it. Emphasis has been on appearance rather than content: white flour, with a host of nutrients removed, processed oils with additives and *orange* oranges, artificially colored, stock the shelves of America's supermarkets. The youngster who lunches on a fast-food hamburger—over 24 billion of them served to date, the sign proclaims—gets a much different diet than did a farm boy whose noon meal consisted of freshly cooked vegetables and meat that wasn't shot full of hormones. We may think we're eating well, but a Harvard University survey reports that the American diet has deteriorated, especially since 1960.

As for the Recommended Daily Allowances (RDA) put forth by the Food and Nutrition Board, they are a *guide* to minimum daily requirements and are woefully low in light of the amounts recommended by many nutrition researchers.

As Senator William Proxmire wrote in *Let's Live,* a health-food magazine: "At best the RDA's are only a 'recommended' allowance at antediluvian levels designed to prevent some terrible disease. At worst, they are based on conflicts of interest and self-serving views of certain parts of the food industry. Almost never are they provided at levels to provide for optimum health and nutrition."

In addition to which, both the RDA and the MDR (Minimum Daily Requirements) are based on the needs of a 22-year-old individual of normal height and weight, living in a temperate climate, wearing proper clothing and engaging in light activity.

The latest information indicates that different individuals have vastly different nutritional needs, so that what may be adequate for one person is sorely lacking for another. Besides these individual differences, age, occupation and stress exert their own nutritional needs.

Although the connection between disease and a deficiency in the diet has long been known, it was not until 1881 that vitamins were discovered. A researcher fed mice a synthetic mixture of the known constituents of milk—protein, fat, carbohydrate and salts—and the mice died. He correctly surmised that milk, a natural food, must contain other substances necessary to life. Some years later they came to be called *vitamins,* from *vita,* Latin for life. These compounds must be manufactured by plants or animals; today, we also manufacture them synthetically in the laboratory, but even there, living organisms are used, similar to the way we make beer or yogurt or cheese.

Among those who agree vitamin supplements are necessary, there is disagreement over whether natural vitamins, from animals or plants, are better than the man-made synthetics. Most nutritionists insist that natural is better, because these vitamins may contain unknown elements that may be important, or may help in the absorption of the desired vitamin. Several studies back up their claims, indicating that synthetic vitamins sometimes have no effect at all until taken in conjunction with the vitamins from natural sources.

The late J. I. Rodale, whose *Prevention* magazine is a Bible to many, tells the story in *The Complete Book of Vitamins* of the attempt to duplicate synthetically sea water for a London aquarium. Several batches were made, but the fish kept dying—until a small amount of real sea water was added. The unknown elements in the actual sea water could not be identified, but obviously they were at work.

Despite the fact that the price of natural or organic vitamins and minerals can be one to five times more than synthetic varieties, we feel that the extra cost is probably justified. We acknowledge that all vitamins have to be chemically extracted from their sources, and that in many cases the organic variety may actually contain a large percentage of the manufactured substance. Nevertheless, inevitably there are minute traces of other substances included in the natural variety, and these may be crucial.

For example, rose hips do not contain enough Vitamin C to make pills of sufficient potency, so Rose Hips Vitamin C—touted and expensive—usually contains some synthetic ascorbic acid (the chemical name of Vitamin C) to boost the strength. However, Vitamin C from natural sources contains a group of substances called *bioflavonoids,* which not only enhance the action of C but also can achieve results that ascorbic acid alone cannot, such as building capillary strength.

What is certain is that borderline deficiencies of vitamins affect the body, although the symptoms might not be as obvious as outright malnutrition. The eyes are sensitive to even slight deficiencies, and depending upon the situation and the stress involved, the amount of vitamins used up by the eyes can vary widely from day to day. There is also some research indicating that some vitamins protect us against the effects of air pollution.

We do not claim to be nutrition experts, but as part of a total approach to vision, we present here some of the current data concerning the relationship of vitamins and minerals to the eyes.

Vitamin A

How often have we heard someone say they do not like driving at night because they have trouble seeing? Or that the glare from the oncoming cars "blinds" them? Or that driving in the dusky light of sunset is the most bothersome? They may be lacking in Vitamin A.

If one estimate is correct, approximately 20 percent of the population have this deficiency. That high figure may be due to one condition of modern life which is difficult to avoid—spending long hours under harsh, glaring lights, which apparently uses up Vitamin A at an accelerated rate. So do polluted air, watching a lot of television, and sports such as skiing and surfing, where one is exposed to sun glare. Driving at night, especially when there are many oncoming headlights, also dips into the body's reserve of A.

The reason this happens is that the ability of the eye to adapt to changes in light is dependent upon a substance called visual purple (technically known as *rhodopsin*). One of the two main components of visual purple is a close relative of Vitamin A. The other is protein. Visual purple surrounds the rods, elongated cells more sensitive to faint light than the more numerous cones, which do most of their work during daylight.

We see an object when light strikes the rods or cones of our retina and is turned into a neural impulse to be sent to the brain, which records the sensation as a visual message. At night, when light is being converted to that electrochemical energy, visual purple breaks up into its components. This occurs, for example, when headlights from an oncoming car come into view. After the car passes, visual purple is reformed. Each time this occurs the body dips into the storeroom for more Vitamin A to regenerate the visual purple. If there isn't enough Vitamin A on hand, this regeneration is slow and imperfect, causing the person to have difficulty adjusting his vision when the illumination changes.

In bright light a similar process takes place in the cone cells, so that a person who suffers from night blindness may also find it necessary to wear sunglasses in bright daylight or be uncommonly uncomfortable without them.

Night blindness can come on slowly, depending on the degree and duration of the Vitamin A deficiency. At first one might only have slight trouble seeing in the dark; then it takes a longer time to adjust to darkness, often noticeable when one enters a darkened movie theater, and eventually, a bright light in the dark—such as a headlight—momentarily leaves one blinded. The eyes can become fatigued easily whenever one attempts to see at night, and there may be dark spots in the field of vision.

Since a deficiency of Vitamin A strips all the mucous membranes of their necessary food, these delicate linings of the eye, throat, intestine, urinary and reproductive tracts dry out and are thus unable to resist the normal invasion of bacteria. The person then becomes highly susceptible to respiratory infections, ranging from tonsilitis to the common cold to pneumonia. Other symptoms of a Vitamin A deficiency include dandruff and rashes; dry, flaky skin and hair, and peeling nails. Nutritionist Adelle Davis and others have reported that people who work under fluorescent lights may suffer from Vitamin A deficiency, and, as a result, are prone to skin blemishes.

Most fluorescent lighting is unhealthy for us anyway, because it lacks the full spectrum of natural daylight, but precisely how it is related to using up large quantities of Vitamin A is not clear. It may be that the flicker of fluorescence is not unlike the off and on glare of oncoming headlights—different in intensity, but sustained over a long period of time.

If the Vitamin A deficiency is allowed to progress unchecked, the eye condition worsens. The problems begin with burning, itching and inflamed eyes, a feeling that one has sand in the eyes; styes may be common. The condition is called conjunctivitis.

Dryness of the cornea—since it is not being effectively lubricated by the tear ducts—can cause spots to appear on its surface. Bitot's spots, named after the physician who first studied them, are triangular, silvery and shiny. Small ulcers may also be noted on the cornea. Untreated, the eye tissues are likely to become so dried out and thickened that the person has *xerophthalmia,* which means, literally, "dry eyes." The tear ducts have simply stopped working. The whole eyeball may run with pus. If the deficiency is not reversed, the ailment can totally destroy the cornea: blindness is the result.

In southern Mexico one out of five children suffers from xerophthalmia, and it can be found among the poor in this country. Before blindness, however, a child often dies from a related disease, such as pneumonia. The sad part of all this is that treatment is so simple and cheap, since Vitamin A is one of our least costly vitamins.

While the average diet in this country provides enough Vitamin A to prevent the more serious diseases, it is generally agreed that we as a nation are not receiving enough for optimal health, especially when one considers the conditions of life today, which seem to demand more. An amount adequate for grandpa, who lived in a small town where the air was not polluted, who did not watch television and who did not work or study under fluorescent lights, does not meet the needs of his grandson who does all of the above. Environment, as we have pointed out before, affects us and changes our needs.

The difficulty with Vitamin A is that there is no general agreement on how much we need. Although the RDA is 5,000 units for adults, 6,000 for pregnant women and 8,000 for nursing women, one of the most respected biochemists working in nutrition, Dr. Roger Williams, states that these figures are no more than an educated guess. And many of us are not even receiving that RDA.

Vitamin A, along with D, E, and K, are oil-soluble vitamins which are stored in body fat. Unlike the water-soluble vitamins (all the rest) they are not quickly washed out of the system. For this reason, an overdose of an oil-soluble vitamin can be troublesome, but it appears that one would need to take massive amounts (100,000 units daily) over a period of months before problems, including drowsiness, headaches, aching bones, nosebleeds and even psychosis, begin. Further, it has been reported that these symptoms cease within a few days or weeks after reducing the amount of Vitamin A.

For most of us, however, the problem is insufficient Vitamin A. Oil-soluble vitamins need the presence of other fats and minerals, and sometimes of one another, to be absorbed properly. Thus a fat-free reducing diet over a long period of time may be dangerous. Oil-soluble vitamins are measured in international units rather than grams, as the water-soluble vitamins are.

Vitamin A is found in greatest quantity in fish, especially the fish-liver oils, from which most capsules are made, and in poultry and animal meats. Liver is the richest source, with two ounces supplying more than 30,000 units, which make the dosages recommended by some vitamin researchers—from 15,000 to 30,000 units daily—seem not out of line. As Vitamin A is contained in fat, whole milk, *not* skim, is a good source, as are egg yolks and butter. Diets designed to eliminate calories and cholesterol may eliminate these sources of A, so supplements of A are often recommended if you are on such a diet.

Carrots and other vegetables do not contain the vitamin itself but a substance called *carotene,* a yellow substance sometimes used to color food, from which the body makes its own Vitamin A. But carotene is stored within the indigestible cell walls and must be released by chopping or chewing or cooking before it can be used by the body. In carrots, less than one percent may actually enter the body, and probably only a small percentage of that is converted to A. To judge from the food pages of magazines and newspapers, the knowledge that "raw is better" is taking America by storm, but that is not true so far as carrots are concerned. Lightly cooked is better.

As for other vegetables, the darker the green or the deeper the yellow, the greater the carotene content, making spinach, beet greens, parsley, watercress, broccoli and the outer leaves of lettuce better choices than paler varieties. Bright yellow apricots are the most concentrated fruit source. Sweet potatoes, turnips, and tomatoes are also rich sources.

How much our food purveyors are sold on the idea that Americans are concerned with appearance rather than nutrition can be told in the story of a tomato developed at Purdue University. The tomatoes had 10 times the Vitamin A content of conventional varieties but were an orange-red color, not the bright red we are used to. They were never marketed, because it was thought the unusual color would be rejected by consumers. The researchers went on to develop a tomato that was a brighter red than most but had approximately half the Vitamin A content of most varieties.

Vitamin A capsules, frequently combined with D (because it occurs naturally that way) are often available in dosages of 5,000 units, which is the RDA. However, even keeping in mind that large amounts of A can be dangerous, the new research indicates that this usually can be stepped up to 15,000 to 30,000 units or more, particularly if there is any indication of eye strain. This means taking three to six capsules daily, preferably spaced throughout the day.

Vitamin A can be destroyed by poor liver function, alcohol, the use of mineral oil, taking ferrous sulfate (a form of iron), X rays, any kind of infection and even cold weather. The carotene in vegetables is extremely susceptible to oxygen, so that 20 minutes after a carrot has been peeled and left sitting on a plate, much of the vitamin has vanished into the air. This is another reason why it is difficult to obtain sufficient vitamins from food.

Recent research indicates that an adequate intake of zinc is crucial to overall health and facilitates the action of many vitamins, including A. One study in Baltimore showed that people with poor night vision— who also had been heavy drinkers for many years—showed no improvement when given supplements of A until 90 milligrams of zinc were given daily. Zinc deficiency can be noted by small white spots under your fingernails.

Because of the inhibiting action of iron on the oil-soluble vitamins, it is best to take them at opposite ends of the day, or at least four hours apart.

The B Vitamins

Fashion aside, if you cannot stand being outdoors in the sunlight —even when it is not too bright—without dark sunglasses, a lack of the B vitamins could be the culprit. Watery eyes, chronic eye fatigue, light sensitivity, burning, bloodshot eyes, twilight blindness and seeing just a part of the page or having dark spots in the field of vision may be related to a lack of this complex family of vitamins—and not just insufficient A. If the problem is acute enough, bits of mucous may collect at the base of the lashes, and during sleep the outer corners of the eyes may crack.

As few as five milligrams of riboflavin—B_2—has been helpful in alleviating these symptoms. Evidence is piling up which indicates a B_2 deficiency may contribute to cataracts, a darkening of the lens. Cataracts, which afflict 75 percent of us over 65, are the leading cause of blindness in the United States.

At the University of Georgia 47 persons with a variety of visual problems, including those mentioned above, were given 15 milligrams of B_2 daily. Some of them reported improvement within a day. Six had cataracts, and after nine months all were reabsorbed; when the B_2 was withdrawn, the cataracts returned until treatment was resumed.

However, if you have cataracts, do not run to the vitamin store and stock up on riboflavin. You will probably end up wondering why your eyes fail to improve. What seems to be helpful in absorbing cataracts is a good diet, supplementary B vitamins—along with others, especially C and E—pantothenic acid (also a B vitamin), minerals and less stress. A new drug is also being tested on animals.

Another example of how the psychological affects the physical is evident in the fact that during times of stress, B vitamins are used up at a rapid rate, since there is a connection between the Bs and the endocrine glands, which regulate the body's machinery.

Dr. Roger Williams, a biologist at the University of Texas, was able to demonstrate that the number of cataracts in laboratory animals are in direct proportion to the lack of certain nutrients in the diet. His findings indicate that when the body is low or completely lacking in the enzyme necessary to metabolize *galactose,* one of the milk sugars, cataracts may result, and that vitamin supplements in the diet may stimulate the body to produce this enzyme. Dr. Williams stresses that his experiments do not prove that one or another vitamin will prevent cataracts, but he suggests that a healthy diet, augmented by vitamins and minerals, may prevent them from forming and help those that are not too advanced to be reabsorbed before surgery is necessary. Other studies over the last quarter of a century back up these findings.

In India, for example, where millions live on meager meals containing few vitamins, cataracts are common early in life; when vitamins (including riboflavin) were given to some, the disease was arrested. In Russia, Vitamin B_{15} in combination with A and E is reported to have dramatic results in treating cataracts and glaucoma; back in the United States, research suggests that the bioflavonoids, substances which are part of the complex Vitamin C found in nature, have the ability to prevent the breakdown of tiny capillary blood vessels, which may be involved in the cataracts developed by so many diabetics.

What all of this adds up to is that while a deficiency of a specific vitamin may appear to be a factor in a specific ailment, the lack of several different nutrients is more likely the culprit. This seems to be especially true in the case of the B vitamins, a family of nutrients always found together in nature. It is generally believed that it is impossible to be deficient in one only, and that if you show glaring deficiencies in one of the Bs, the others are probably not far behind. In fact, taking one of the B vitamins alone usually increases the need for others not supplied; over a long period of time, high doses of a particular B may produce problems which do more harm than the good for which they were intended.

Sometimes, however, specific ailments are associated with a deficiency of one or more of the Bs. For one example, insufficient thiamin (B_1) can cause pains behind the eyeball, and a serious lack of the vitamin may lead to paralysis of the eye muscle.

The Bs are often able to alleviate diseases which affect the eyes. Meniere's disease, an illness causing mental disturbances, and pellegra, which killed approximately 10,000 victims a year at the turn of the century, have serious eye implications. Both diseases respond to B vitamins: Meniere's to the complex, and pellegra to niacin, a vitamin that is lost in the refining process of cornmeal, a staple of the Southern diet where the disease can still be found among the poor. Some types of pellegra, in which there is a loss of eyelashes, inflammation of the eyelids, and general erosion of tissue, will not respond to niacin alone, and other members of the B complex are needed.

One of the consequences of smoking is that inordinate amounts of B_{12} are destroyed by the tars and nicotine, and the result may be a dimming of vision. A person may complain that he is having trouble reading, or tires quickly. What happens is that the constituents of tobacco decompose the myelin sheaths protecting the nerve endings, and the optic nerve is the first to be affected. A person suffering from *tobacco amblyopia* may also have frequent headaches, blackouts, cold fingertips in the morning after that first cigarette, and difficulty in discerning green and red. When the individual stops smoking, vision often quickly returns to normal. If B_{12} is given early enough and the nerve has not deteriorated, complete recovery is possible.

Cigar and pipe smokers are in just as much difficulty here as cigarette smokers. And even constantly being in the presence of smokers can be hazardous, making the trend to prohibit smoking in public places, such as elevators, sections of restaurants and airplanes—and even some newspaper cityrooms—all the more welcome. To nonsmokers.

According to the latest research we are not getting sufficient Bs in our diet; a 1969 investigation of preschool children revealed that 21 percent were suffering from a B_2 deficiency. At least part of the reason is that the white flour we use has most of these nutrients processed out of it and left on the milling room floor. "Refortified" white bread is still seriously lacking in them.

In addition, our poor eating habits seem designed to require high quantities of the Bs. Coffee, sugar—the consumption of which continues to rise due to our predilection for pastry, soft drinks, and ice cream—and alcohol gobble up the Bs. Alcohol also washes them out of the body; this relationship led Navy researchers to conclude during World War II that munching on Bs rather than peanuts might prevent a hangover.

The Bs are water-soluble vitamins, making them readily absorbed in the body and just as readily washed out, so that a new supply should be coming in daily. Since they are not stored to any great extent in the body, you need not worry about getting too much of a good thing —unless you overdose on a single one of the family. Like C, another water-soluble vitamin, they are measured in milligrams and grams.

How much do you need? The answer depends on how big you are —how many cells do you have to feed? How much alcohol and coffee do you drink? How much sugar and processed food do you eat? Some people have noted that the craving for sugar can be somewhat controlled by taking plenty of B complex.

The foods rich in Vitamin B are liver, eggs, whole grains, nuts and sunflower seeds. Among members of the natural-food set sunflower seeds enjoy a lofty reputation as a wonder food for almost everything— eyes, nerves, energy. They do contain a stockpile of all kinds of nutrients and are especially high in the Bs. Of course they should be purchased unhulled and untoasted; you do the hulling yourself and eat them raw. Chew well.

Leafy green vegetables, fruits and meat also contain the Bs, but because these vitamins are not very stable, exposure to light, air and water can make them vanish into the atmosphere or down the drain— if you throw out the cooking water.

Brewer's yeast, a natural food containing at least 10 of the known members of the rambling B family, is prized by vitamin aficionados. It can be mixed into milk or fruit juices, but, yes, it does somewhat alter the taste. Some people say you get to like it after a while; it may be a question of mind over matter, if you keep telling yourself how good it is for you. You might try brewer's yeast pills instead.

Wheat germ is another good source. This can be eaten by itself as a cereal or mixed with others, sprinkled on fruits, vegetables and yogurt, and added to some recipes.

If you are going to take B complex capsules, make sure they provide more than minute traces of the vitamins. Most nutritionists suggest taking pills containing at least 50 milligrams of several of the components, and spacing them throughout the day, particularly after a meal or snack, which is the best time to take any vitamin.

If you have been low in the Bs, your body will let you know in a big way as soon as you start taking them: temporary fullness, gas and weight gain are the signals. Retreat a bit and lower your dosage for a while. With brewer's yeast, start out with a half-teaspoon daily for a week, then go on to a whole teaspoon, gradually increasing up to a few tablespoons daily.

Vitamin C

Vitamin C and the Common Cold, a slim volume by Dr. Linus Pauling, set off a controversy in 1970 which has not yet been settled, even though the evidence continues to mount that megadoses of this vitamin—the only one which our body cannot produce on its own from other nutrients—not only help to prevent colds and other infections, but also hasten their departure.

Vitamin C is the substance which carries hydrogen to all the cells of our body. It is necessary to convert food into energy. Vitamin C has a special function in the white blood cells, which fight infection, and is suspected of actually stripping viruses of their potency. Other research indicates it protects cells from the onslaught of air and water pollution. It is an ingredient the body uses to manufacture collagen, the binding substance that holds our cells and bones together. Understanding that the health of our eyes is closely linked with our general health, it is no surprise that adequate C may be crucial to the eye.

The healthy lens of the eye is rich in this vitamin, while the diseased lens contains little or none. Glaucoma and cataracts are accompanied by low levels of C in the lens, which apparently relates to the fact that older people, who are susceptible to these ailments, are often especially deficient in Vitamin C. Not only does it appear that older folks might need more C than youngsters, but due to changes in life style and diet, they may actually be getting less. A mother who insists that her children drink orange juice at breakfast and eat lots of leafy green vegetables at dinner may neglect to follow this dictum when she is a widow living alone. Her income may be lower, as well as her interest in food. Cooking for one is not the same as planning a family meal.

In any event, the dosages of C which the new research suggests far exceed what we can get through food. The recommendations: 1 to 5 grams daily, and up to 10 at the first sign of a sniffle. Remember that an orange averages 60 milligrams of C—not grams, milligrams. That's 1/1000th of a gram.

There is some evidence that Vitamin C may be effective in treating glaucoma, which afflicts more than two million Americans and is a major cause of blindness. At least a quarter of a million people in this country have lost the sight of one eye due to glaucoma. The pressure at the back of the eyeball increases due to an abnormal amount of fluid; as it does so, the optic nerve is pushed back toward the brain, distorting vision and possibly closing off the tiny drainage canal at the front of the eye. The optic nerve and retina may eventually be destroyed by the pressure, and when that happens, sight goes too. There is no cure, only several methods of controlling glaucoma: eye drops, drugs (some with adverse side effects), and surgery in the advanced cases. Currently, marijuana is being investigated, with encouraging results to date. The drug is either smoked or applied topically.

In a test at the University of Rome doctors prescribed large doses of Vitamin C to patients with severe glaucoma. The doses were individualized according to body weight. A person weighing 150 pounds would receive 35 grams daily—far more than the megadoses taken by some to ward off colds—and the results were a rapid and significant drop in intraocular pressure, with the lowest pressure in the eye when the level of C in the bloodstream was the highest. The dosage had to be spaced throughout the day to prevent stomach upset, but otherwise there were no side effects.

Other researchers have found that large amounts of C may possibly prevent cataracts in diabetics, who are unusually prone to them. A British study reports that the healing of corneal ulcers appears to be hastened by taking 1,500 milligrams of C daily.

Since C helps to keep capillaries, the tiniest blood vessels, functioning in top form, they are less likely to break down and cause a slight hemorrhage, which often is seen as a bruise. People whose gums bleed easily (a minor hemorrhage) or wonder where they got all those bruises often find these conditions are alleviated when supplementary C is taken. This safety measure against hemorrhaging obviously extends to the eyes. In scurvy, a disease that is virtually nonexistent today because we generally have some C in our diet, there are hemorrhages of the eyelids and eye tissues. The treatment for scurvy since 1600 has been Vitamin C—and even a trace of it is adequate. There is enough C in a blade of grass to cure scurvy, which shows how tiny an amount is crucial to health and how important vitamins are.

The best food sources of C are the citrus fruits—oranges, grapefruits, lemons, and limes—but up to 40 percent of their vitamin content may be lost in a month's storage. The peels of these fruits, ounce for ounce, are two or three times as potent as the juice—but not when they are cooked for marmalade. Tomato juice, fresh or canned, has approximately half as much C as the citrus juices. Most fresh fruits contain some, but the amount varies widely from fruit to fruit. Apples are low (and, again, most is lost during long storage) and berries are high. Melons are good sources, considering the size of an ordinary serving.

Most vegetables contain C, but how they are cooked determines how much we get. A baked potato contains approximately 20 milligrams, but french fries contain practically none. Cabbage, cooked quickly and eaten immediately, is a good source; so are brussels sprouts. Watercress, ounce for ounce, is more potent than orange juice, but we do not consume more than a few ounces of this green in a typical salad. However, as head lettuce contains almost no C, it would be worth switching from lettuce to cress as a staple in our salads.

Vitamin C is the most unstable of all vitamins, and a great deal is lost in the way we prepare our food. Soaking cabbage to "crisp" it reduces its C content to nearly nothing. To retain as much as possible, vegetables should be cooked in a steamer or in a small amount of water for the shortest possible time needed to make them palatable. Even with this care, perhaps a fourth of the Vitamin C will be left in the cooking water—along with other vitamins and minerals. This is why the water should be saved for soups, gravies or other recipes calling for liquids.

Raw is best, but even here, exposure to air destroys the vitamin; it is best to chop, slice or shred just before serving. If you cannot, at least store the vegetables in the refrigerator in an air-tight container. As a final caution, adding baking soda to the cooking water for a nice bright color destroys C, and, interestingly, so does cooking in copper pots and pans.

C is another water-soluble vitamin which is not stored in the body and so must be constantly replaced; excess amounts are released in the urine. Vitamin C is rapidly used up by smoking—each cigarette steals approximately 25 milligrams from the body. Stress—anything from having a fight with your mate to an overdue bill—also depletes our stock of C, as do drugs such as cortisone, antibiotics and sulfa.

The C vitamin, like the others, is best taken after meals, not only so that most of it is absorbed but to eliminate stomach distress due to the acid content. Diabetics taking insulin should have medical supervision when starting a Vitamin C regimen, because the vitamin increases the efficiency of insulin and may disrupt the sugar-insulin balance.

There are two forms of Vitamin C: the entire family known as the bioflavonoids, and ascorbic acid. Synthetic ascorbic acid, much cheaper than the natural compound, is what Linus Pauling suggests taking. There are some indications, however, that C in the complex form works synergistically and can accomplish results that ascorbic acid alone cannot.

Some research suggests that bioflavonoids may be helpful in preventing cataracts related to diabetes, which appear to be caused by excessive glucose in the blood reacting with an enzyme. In the test tube, at least, the bioflavonoids prevented the appearance of the troublesome enzyme.

The bioflavonoids, sometimes called Vitamin P, are found naturally in red peppers, the white membrane of citrus fruits and in high amounts in acerola cherries and rose hips, which brings us back to why Rose Hips Vitamin C is prized. Of the two forms of C—bioflavonoids and ascorbic acid, which is best? It depends. Bioflavonoids work more slowly and appear to be the crucial agent in strengthening capillaries. Ascorbic acid in massive amounts is more effective in an emergency, such as the onset of a cold. Some nutritionists and doctors prescribe both.

Bioflavonoids are sometimes sold separately under the name CPR, for Vitamin C, P for the bioflavonoids, and R for rutin, also a factor in the bioflavonoids.

Rutin, in fact, has been credited as the critical agent in strengthening capillaries. Since these crisscross the eye, it follows that their condition will reflect upon its general health. It is worth noting that one common condition in which the tiny blood vessels can be seen to be out of order is diabetes, and in its advanced stage this disease is generally accompanied by cataracts.

Because rutin strengthens blood vessels, it appears to be helpful for people with high blood pressure since it allows the capillaries to withstand greater pressure and thereby reduces the possibility of stroke.

While rutin does not lower blood pressure, it does appear to reduce the pressure in the eye of a person suffering from glaucoma. In one trial of 26 persons, a drop in interocular pressure was noted in 17 patients who were given 20 milligrams three times a day.

One of the richest sources of rutin is buckwheat, an item not found on many grocery lists these days. Even if it were you would have to eat it quickly, for as the buckwheat dries the rutin evaporates. As for other sources, you can hardly beat rose hips.

Because the bioflavonoids, of which rutin is one, are not stored in the body, you cannot overdose. Suggested daily supplements range from 20 milligrams to 1 gram, depending on need. If you bruise easily, have diabetes, high blood pressure or catch colds frequently, some nutritionists suggest the higher dosages or Vitamin C tablets prepared with rose hips. Some of the new preparations list the amount of bioflavonoids included.

Vitamin D and Calcium

Although Vitamin A is usually called the Eye Vitamin, a New York City ophthalmologist reserves that title for D, the one we absorb from sunlight. Dr. Arthur Knapp has successfully treated a number of eye ailments—including myopia—with D and calcium. In some cases acuity was more than doubled, Dr. Knapp wrote in the *Journal of the International Academy of Preventive Medicine.* Thus a person with 20/400 acuity (20/200 *with glasses* is considered legal blindness) improved to 20/200—or better.

In treating patients whose myopia was increasing rapidly, over 50 percent showed a change for the better, Dr. Knapp reported. Some remained the same—in contrast to the further deterioration expected— and a full third showed an actual reduction in myopia.

In trials at Columbia's College of Physicians and Surgeons, animals fed diets deficient in Vitamin D and calcium developed a wide range of eye problems as well as arteriosclerosis, a clogging of the arteries that interferes with blood circulation.

Dr. Knapp then gave D and calcium to humans suffering from several eye ailments—keratoconus (a protrusion of the cornea); cataract; retinitis pigmentosa (a degenerative disease which leads to night blindness); detached retina; glaucoma, and myopia. The results were a significant improvement in a high percentage of cases. The vitamin and calcium go together, because D is needed for the proper absorption of calcium, which gives us strong bones and muscles, the eye muscles included. Several other studies show that the myopic child is frequently deficient in calcium.

In the case of myopia, the vitamin and mineral combination appears to change the fibrous tunic surrounding the eyeball by dehydrating it. If this shell is waterlogged, it seems to be susceptible to the pressure within and stretches into the elongated shape of a nearsighted eye. By dehydrating this tunic, the eyeball actually shrinks back to the more normal shape, thereby reducing the myopia.

For some of the conditions reported by Dr. Knapp, the dosage was 50,000 units of D daily—given for an indeterminate period of time —and one gram of calcium. This treatment should only be taken under strict medical supervision, of course.

Another researcher, working independently 30 years ago, also credits a build up of water pressure in the eye as a prime factor leading to nearsightedness. Dr. Hunter Turner blamed the high consumption of carbonated beverages for a waterlogging of the entire body. In the stomach the carbonated drinks break down into their basic ingredients of water and carbon dioxide, which travel to every part of the body; this means that an abnormal amount of water is trapped in the eye tissues and constricts their smooth and easy functioning.

Soft drinks also pour a lot of sugar down the throat, and sugar is at least coincidentally related to the incidence of myopia, as we will soon discuss.

Sunshine is our main source of D. Its ultraviolet rays must penetrate the lower layer of the skin to activate the production of D. Consequently, dark-skinned people are more likely to be deficient in D than pale folk, and rickets (a softening of bone tissue) is more common among black children than white. Dark tans, status symbol though they be, also limit our ability to absorb D.

A noontime sitting in the sun with exposed face, neck, and arms provides a useful amount. Smog and fog naturally reduce the amount of D which reaches us.

We can get some Vitamin D through fish, egg yolk, milk, and butter, but the amount is negligible. Milk fortified with Vitamin D is good, but even a quart a day does not provide enough.

The best supplemental sources are fish-oil capsules (especially halibut), and D usually comes in combination with A, as they are found together in nature. In tandem—with a little help from C—they are useful in preventing colds.

Cod liver oil, the old standby which made some of us gag as kids, fortunately has been replaced by the capsules. Sometimes the oil-soluble vitamins (of which D is one) are defatted and sold in other preparations, and these can be more quickly absorbed, but the vitamins do not function as well as when taken in their natural state.

How much do we need? Again, no one is sure. Like A, Vitamin D is stored in the body, and an overdose can be toxic, causing much the same symptoms as too much A. But the literature indicates that problems do not begin until one takes 50,000 units daily for weeks. Since the highest potency D capsules commonly available have 5,000 international units, you would have to take 10 a day to reach the danger zone. The newer vitamin regimens call for between 800 and 1,200 units daily.

Expectant and nursing mothers should be sure to get adequate D, since the child, before and after birth, needs D to process calcium and phosphate for strong bones and teeth. A large amount of these minerals pass out through mother's milk, and when she does not obtain enough from her food or supplements, her bones and teeth give them up. It has been suggested that expectant mothers take a supplement of 1,000 to 2,000 units daily, in addition to drinking a quart of whole milk. Skim milk may have fewer calories—but it also has fewer vitamins.

Vitamin E

The glamour vitamin of the last decade has been E, which has been credited with doing just about everything: dissolve blood clots, promote healing of wounds and reducing scars, improve circulation, lessen leg cramps, retard aging of the cells, keep our hearts in good working order—and doesn't it have something to do with sexuality?

Well, it has been shown that laboratory animals on diets deficient in E can conceive but not carry the fetus to delivery. Among women patients it also appears that Vitamin E can help prevent miscarriage. The vitamin is apparently needed by the body to manufacture the substance that binds the growing embryo to the wall of the uterus throughout pregnancy. In fact, the chemical name for Vitamin E is tocopherol, which comes from the Greek words meaning *child* and *to bear*.

Some claim that Vitamin E will alleviate impotency; what we know for sure is that its lack in animals leads to sterility. The placebo effect may have a lot to do with its reputation for enhancing sexuality in humans—if you think a substance is an aphrodisiac, it may well prove to be.

Because the claims made for Vitamin E are so numerous, many doubt that it could work such wonders, but the evidence continues to mount that E may indeed be deserving of its reputation. It is possible it works in so many ways because it increases the ability of the veins and arteries to carry oxygen, and since these pathways go everywhere, the salubrious effects of increased oxygenation do also. Vitamin E also has been shown to increase the effectiveness of the other vitamins, notably A and C, which, as we have seen, are crucial to general well-being.

The many benefits of Vitamin E naturally extend to the eyes. In animal tests its lack in the diet caused clouding of the cornea, cataracts and other abnormalities of the retina and lens. It has been shown to be effective in treating a number of human eye diseases when taken over a period of months. In a 1953 Italian study with 400 patients, the doctors conducting the study reported uniformly good results for a wide variety of eye ailments; in some cases even improved acuity was noted.

Vitamin E has been shown to enable new blood vessels to form, and this may be at least partly responsible for the fact that it appears to be extremely helpful in arresting—or even reversing—the degenerative changes in the eyes which normally come with old age. In another Italian study, patients over 40 years old were given Vitamin E, and their presbyopia was reduced to the point where they could once again read without glasses. In yet another study with patients who had limited degeneration of certain parts of the eye, and thus saw with "blind" spots, the majority showed a reduction of the spots and a rapid return of better vision.

Two French doctors working more than two decades ago, when little was known about E's role in human nutrition, were able to halt the progression of myopia among young patients. Vitamin E has a salubrious effect on connective tissue, or collagen. The doctors proposed that when the collagen fibers of the eyes lose their elasticity they cannot give the support needed to keep the eye from assuming an abnormal shape if other factors—such as too much near-point work—are putting stress on the eye.

The treatment they devised (50-100 milligrams daily) would be considered low by current standards, but even so they found that E taken over a decade generally prevented their patients from becoming more nearsighted.

The leafy green vegetables—lettuce, spinach, watercress and the rest—have an abundance of E, but the food richest in E is wheat germ— that part of the wheat which is discarded when wheat is milled into white flour. However, even eating pounds of wheat germ daily would not bring the E intake up to where it would have the effects we are talking about. Except for those with high blood pressure or rheumatic heart conditions, megadoses of E appear to be nontoxic. What does seem evident, however, is that taking half as much as you need does not do half the job.

Recommended dosages for E usually start with 100 or 200 I.U.s daily, with gradual increases each week. The suggested daily intake varies from 300 to 1,200 units (and higher in some cases), depending on the circumstances and the individual. Nutritionists often recommend setting your own level where results are evident, but by now, if you have been taking the other vitamins, it will obviously be difficult to determine which is doing what. Remember that all vitamins and minerals work synergistically, with calcium helping D and E giving C a hand, and so on. What matters is feeling good and seeing clearly.

Protein

We all know that protein is necessary for strength and vitality. In fact, its Greek root means "of first importance," and its connection with eyesight may be of that order. Almost 20 years ago a British study found a strong relationship between the progression of nearsightedness in children and the amount of protein in the diet. Myopia generally starts in childhood and progresses until the age of 20 or so.

Half of the children in the group had their diet altered so that 10 percent of their normal caloric intake consisted of animal protein; the other half was given no dietary advice. Some of the children over 12 in the special diet group showed a definite arresting of myopia. In others the condition actually reversed itself to some degree. For children under 12 the results were less spectacular but still encouraging: while their eyesight continued to deteriorate, the rate of change was slowed by two-thirds. Those who had the most protein showed the least progression of myopia.

The study also found that myopia is greater and more prevalent among children who refuse to eat animal protein than among those who like their hamburgers, fried chicken and steak. The nearsighted children whose vision was deteriorating ate less food—yet gained more weight—than the children with healthy vision. It could be that children who become nearsighted have metabolic disorders which prevent the proper transformation of food into fuel for the body. Some suggest that protein foods contain enzymes necessary to process food, and that these are found in lesser quantities or are not present at all in the junk foods too many of us consume.

Sugar

If nutritionists were asked to name the scourge of the Western diet, most of them would put sugar at the head of the list. In recent years refined sugar has been blamed for everything from dandruff to diabetes. New evidence relates diabetes to the disruption of the orderly metabolic process brought about by refined sugar, and, as we know, diabetes is often accompanied by cataracts.

Per capita, we Americans consume approximately 70 pounds of sugar a year—and the Germans and English eat even more. It is found in everything from peanut butter to frozen vegetables, not just in cakes, colas and candy bars. It's actually added to some brands of table salt. One popular burger chain puts seven times the normal amount of sugar in its buns, and America is gobbling them up at the rate of billions each year.

Refined sugar, in contrast to the fructose found naturally in fruit, consumes huge quantities of vitamins and minerals, particularly calcium, sodium and phosphorus, as the sugar is processed in the body. The healthy eye needs the whole gamut of these vitamins and minerals for good living, just as the rest of the body needs them.

One Japanese researcher believes that diet, along with other environmental factors, plays a major role in myopia. "If you give sugar to a rabbit, the rabbit becomes myopic," is the blunt way Dr. Jin Otsuka puts it. He relates the rise and fall of the incidence of myopia in Japan before and after World War II with the rise and fall of the supply of sugar and other refined foods. The more sugar in the diet, the greater the incidence of myopia. During the war years the Japanese returned to their traditional rice and fish diet, and myopia plummeted. However, this observation does not take into consideration another factor: the war disrupted the school system, so young people were not putting in long hours of study at near point, which appears to be closely related to the amount of myopia.

The same connection between diet and eye disease is found in several other studies, including ones among the Eskimos of Alaska, the aborigines of Australia and British school children. A 1977 study reported in the *Canadian Journal of Public Health* relates the amount of myopia in the Amerind Indians of northern Ontario to the lack of animal protein in their diet. It notes that the Eskimos of Belcher Island, while from a different genetic pool, have more access to fish and game and have significantly less myopia than the Amerinds, even though the two groups have a basically similar life style.

Although each vitamin and mineral has its own job to do, it is their combined action which promotes the normal and healthy operating of the body—and the eye. The intelligent nutritional approach is one which takes this synergism into consideration and does not, for example, load up on A and E, while forgetting about zinc: all the elements work better with a little help from their friends. Teamwork is the key.

And it appears that a high intake of refined sugar makes the job that much more difficult, since it burns up so many perfectly good vitamins and minerals just as they are being processed in the body.

We of course are not saying that supernutrition will let you throw away your glasses, but it does appear that it can be extremely beneficial in warding off—and in some cases, actually healing—eye ailments.

We know that many persons will remain unconvinced that vitamins should be taken in the form of supplements. "I eat well—my grandfather lived to be a hundred and he didn't take them." But your grandfather probably did not live in a smog-saturated city, work under fluorescent lights, watch television or drive a car at night. It's possible that your grandfather didn't go to college nor was he highly anxious about getting good grades—factors which overload our eyes with stress. Certainly, he didn't eat convenience foods with much of their nutrients processed out and the flavor restored with artificial flavorings and additives. The vitamin content of a baked potato is vastly different from what you'll get in most restaurants when you order "mashed" potatoes. Often these are the reconstituted dehydrated variety, since only the educated palate can tell the difference once they are laden with butter or gravy.

In addition to which, all the evidence points to the fact that supernutrition—good food supplemented with extra vitamins and minerals—is the road to super health. The more research is done, the more we are aware that these substances can work seeming miracles. A whole branch of therapy—orthomolecular or, as it is more commonly called, megavitamin—has grown up around this premise.

By supplementing psychotherapy and drugs with high doses of vitamins and minerals, several doctors are achieving spectacular results. Dr. David Hawkins of the North Nassau Mental Health Clinic in Manhasset, Long Island, says that in treating schizophrenia he can just about double the recovery rate, halve the rehospitalization rate and virtually eliminate self-destruction in a disease whose victims experience a suicide rate 22 times that of the general population. Dr. Allan Cott, a New York City psychiatrist, reports dramatic success by treating children who are autistic or have other learning disabilities with high doses of vitamins. Megavitamin therapy has also been used to treat alcoholism, drug conditions, senility and infant psychosis, in addition to depression and schizophrenia.

Visual distortion is one of the first clues that something is wrong mentally, and in the written personality test given to many mental patients before treatment begins, the first section has such questions as: "Do people's faces sometimes look strange? Does yours in a mirror? Do words look funny on the page? Do you see haloes? Do objects seem to move? Do you see animals that others do not? Do words move around when you read? Does the picture on television ever look strange? Do objects seem to pulsate when you look at them? Do you see sparks in front of you?"

If vision is not intimately tied to the brain and our perception of the world, why do the mentally disturbed see peculiarly? The evidence that the eye and the brain operate as a unit has been there all along. We have until now chosen to ignore it.

7
Maintaining Good Vision

*But if, realizing the situation, we compose ourselves and de-
cide not to continue, everything will right itself in time.*

If men today, as Dorothy Parker wrote, don't make passes at girls
who wear glasses, their pickings are slim. Approximately 50 percent of
our population wears glasses.

Fortunately for this multitude, glasses have been turned into a
fashion accessory: tortoise frames, wire frames, red, white and blue
frames. You can have them big or small, round or oblong or square.
The lenses can be clear or rose-colored or designed to lighten and
darken as the day does. Rock stars wear heart-shaped frames, and the
society dame has diamonds in hers for nights at the opera.

But why are so many of us walking around in specs? After millions of years of evolution, why are our eyes breaking down at such a
rate? The trouble usually begins to be noticed during the early school
years and the percentages rise steadily with more education. If you look
at it one way, you could say that intelligence is related to weak eyes.
That would be erroneous, of course, but what's happening is that the
pursuit of knowledge often puts the eyes under a strain that results in
visual problems.

But it need not be so.

Only 2 or 3 percent of the population have eye problems at birth,
yet possibly a full 70 percent run into some kind of trouble with sight
during their lifetimes. In addition to the obvious problems, such as nearsightedness, farsightedness and astigmatism, there are those we don't
know we have but which keep us from operating at top performance:
trouble tracking a line across a page, shifting focus from far to near,
difficulty converging on an object. Some of us don't use both eyes together, but only one at a time.

The question is: what are we doing to ourselves to wear out our eyes while the rest of the machine is still going strong? You are doing it right this minute as you concentrate on little black marks on a page, which you translate into meaning. Now there's nothing wrong with that —it's doing it hour after hour without respite that is the problem. Man's eyes evolved to direct us as we walked through the forests and over mountains, trapping animals and planting grain. Eyes were made to look at sunsets and horizons. These days we barely give them a chance to do anything but concentrate on details.

The average high school student will plow through some 432 books in 12 years, 36 a year. In college that number jumps to 51 a year, according to one survey. Which gives little time for eyes to do what they do best: look off toward the horizon.

You won't get good grades by doing that, and even after you've graduated and landed that job on Wall Street or have opened up shop as a doctor, your life will be filled with tiny calibrations and intense concentration. The broker will read ticker tape and columns of numbers; the doctor will have to make time at night to plow through the journals if he's going to stay on top of what's happening in his field; the fabric designer will spend her days working on intricate patterns.

What has happened is that the level of work we are asking of our eyes is greater than what they were made to handle. And like an overworked radiator in a car caught in stop-and-go traffic, they break down. Glasses have become the badge of courage handed the child who chooses to push through the massive amount of material society expects him to digest. Dyslexia and juvenile delinquency may be the escape hatches for the child who simply gives up.

Now several things occur when we ask the mind to be alert and think critically: our muscles tense, our breathing gets shallow. We adapt our whole body into a *fight* posture. *The book may be difficult, but I'll get through it,* we consciously or unconsciously tell ourselves.

And later, when we end up with a sore back, we don't feel like taking time out to run a mile or go out for the basketball team. In effect, the body says: *Are you crazy? I'm tired and I just want some time off* . . . and we end up giving the eyes neither, but relax by watching television or reading a magazine article on how to plant petunias in a window box. The material is not as difficult, but we're still looking at little marks on a page or just sitting without moving.

There has been a physical reaction to this sedentary state of affairs. Well-being through exercise has practically become a national preoccupation, and health clubs and spas have sprung up coast to coast.

Tens of thousands have become serious joggers. Massage and movement therapies have gained acceptance and popularity. The name of a good masseuse who'll come to your home is shared with friends over lunches of Perrier water and broiled fish, plain, at the Polo Lounge and Palm Court.

How much we learn through reading is directly related to how efficiently our eyes operate. The more demanding the concentration, the greater degree of efficiency the eyes must have.

We can't avoid all the reading that is required today, but we can make life a little easier for our eyes. It may seem like a waste of time to look out the window every so often, but in the end you may not get as tired; you may be able to absorb more, and maybe you won't push your eyes past the point where there is nothing they can do except adapt to the strain they're under, and so give you trouble when you want to do something else. Like see clearly at a hundred feet or play tennis or shoot ducks.

Perhaps the single most important factor in protecting your eyes when you read is to take a break approximately every 20 minutes. For the average reader, that will be every 15 or 20 pages. Look up across the room or out the window at a distance of 10 or 15 feet away. Refocus your eyes on a small object across the room. The object should be as clear as when you first started reading. If not, do not continue until it does become clear.

To hasten clarity, look at a word in this book for a count of three, look across the room at the object for another count of three, back to the book, up to the object, until the image is clear. Shifting the focus back and forth for a few minutes should chase away the fuzz.

Or you might take a short break. Stand up and stretch. Move around. Try to press your shoulder blades back as if you could make them touch. But do not go on reading until the distant focus is as clear as the printed page was before you started to read.

After an hour of sitting, get up and move. The eyes should not be focused for close work for more than 20 minutes, and the body should not be restricted and sedentary for more than an hour.

While reading or writing, make sure that you are breathing properly. If your breathing is shallow, try some deep breathing for a minute or two.

Also, do not block out peripheral vision, a common practice of people who get too involved in close, detailed work. Try not to be distracted, but be aware of what is going on around you without having to focus on it. People who block out peripheral vision tend to lose the ability to see what's going on outside a narrow and limited perspective, and this may come to be how they relate to the world.

Posture

When reading or writing, you should be seated at a desk in a comfortable chair, not lying on your stomach or on your side. Which is why reading in bed—a favorite pastime of millions—is almost never a

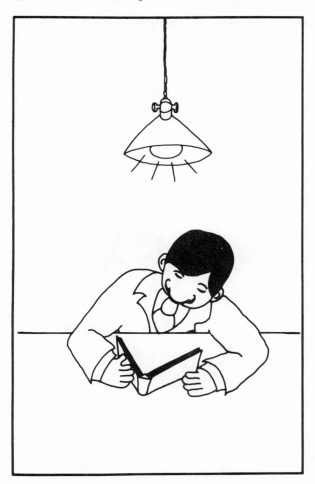

When the back is consistently scrunched over or propped up with one arm, the poor posture that results can lead to poor vision.

good idea. Your back should have a normal curve of the spine, and not be scrunched over or propped up with one arm. If continued long enough, especially by children, the reading position in bed becomes the normal one, and sitting in a chair at a desk becomes abnormal. The visual system gets used to operating from a distorted perspective.

An extra word of caution is added here: try not to read when you're sick. Your eyes are particularly vulnerable and will be more

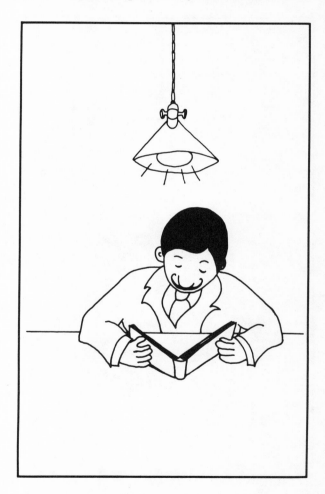

Good posture is when the back follows the normal curve of the spine.

likely to adapt to the warped posture you assume while abed for long periods of time. Consequently, they may not be able to straighten out when you are no longer lying down and want your normal perspective back. Reading may keep you from being bored while you're bedridden, but while you are giving your body a break, include your eyes.

Now that we've got you in a chair, let's consider what kind it should be. It should permit the feet to be flat on the floor; if the feet do not touch, use a phone book or a box under them. The lower back should be supported. The desk or table should be at waist level when the person is seated. Working at a surface too high gives as much distortion as viewing a movie from front row, far side.

The material you are looking at should be in front of the eyes, and at a distance equal to the distance measured between your knuckles and your elbows. To measure this, hold the material in front of you so that your elbow makes a right angle when you're holding the book.

The incline of the book is also important. The text should be parallel to the plane of your face, not flat on the desk, which is why desks constructed at a 20 degree incline are better for reading and writing than flat surfaces.

The parents of a scholar—or anyone who reads and writes a great deal—should consider constructing a simple inclined platform to set on a desk. Yes, it seems like a great deal of bother—and you have gotten by all these years, haven't you? But answer this: Do you wear glasses? Do you tire fast? Would you like to be able to read more efficiently with less effort? Flat surfaces cause the visual system to work harder to make up for the distortion.

If you hold the book you are reading, don't let it lie on your lap—hold it up so the page is parallel with the plane of your face.

Any postural imbalance throws the whole body out of kilter, and the eyes attempt to make up for what's askew. In the process, they may see in a distorted manner. If kept up long enough, the eyes could end up with problems such as astigmatism or one eye tending to drift upward more than the other.

Lighting

Besides furniture, lighting is the other critical factor in determining posture, for a person will unconsciously shift his position to accommodate illumination. If he sees a glare out of the corner of his eye, the individual will shift his head and body to block the distracting center of brightness.

Overhead lighting, which illuminates the whole room or work space, is extremely important in making life easier while reading. The eyes respond to contrast, and a single source of light in a dark room provides just that. Because of the sharp differences in the light intensities, the eyes have to overwork, causing difficulty in concentration. The source of the light is unconsciously distracting the eyes while the mind is consciously trying to attend to the book. Studying in a darkened room under a desk lamp is asking the eyes to work against themselves.

For the same reason, try to avoid writing on white paper on a dark desk. Although deep-toned desks are popular, they add more strain to the eyes, which constantly adjust to the difference between the white paper and dark finish. If you do have such a dark desk, use a blotting pad of medium tone under the paper to cut down on the contrast at the edge of the paper.

While you may not want to take down those Indian bedspreads from which you have made a tent in your living room, give some consideration to the wall colors—and your eyes—in areas where a lot of close work will be done, not only reading but sewing, carpentry, painting or hooking rugs. Soft colors and matte finishes are best. Again, avoid sharp contrasts of colors which fight for your attention, even when you think you are concentrating on the task at hand. It's like trying to study Latin declensions in a room where rock music is blaring. Probably it can be done, but with a great deal of difficulty. You wouldn't try to read Homer in a disco, so why should your eyes have to put up with visual interferences?

In addition to overhead lighting, supplementary lighting for the specific task is desirable. The bulb should be shaded so that the eye isn't exposed to the direct light. If a standing lamp is used, place it approximately two feet behind the text and a little more than a foot to the side of the reader's shoulder. Unless your walls are covered in brown suede, a 150-watt bulb should suffice. If you are using a lamp on a table next to your chair, place it off your shoulder—right or left—and use at least a 100-watt bulb. If you have a desk or gooseneck lamp, use a 75-watt bulb and place the fixture about a foot above the book.

The amount of needed illumination will vary with the depth of the color of the walls. Darker colors absorb more light than paler walls. If you paint or paper your walls a darker tone, you'll easily notice the difference in the amount of light the old bulbs give in the same room. As a general principle, in an average-size room with light-toned walls, the overhead lighting should be between 150 to 200 watts, and the supple-

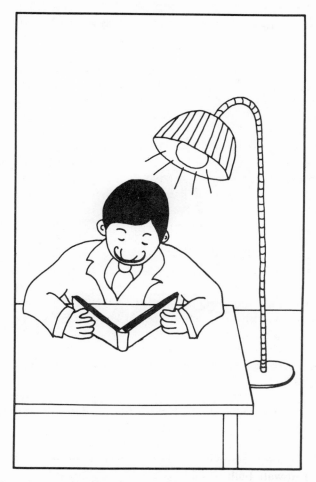

A floor lamp with a 150-watt bulb placed two feet behind the book and one foot to the side should provide good supplementary lighting.

mentary lighting from 75 to 150 watts. The best rule of thumb is that no part of the room should be in darkness.

While intensity and location of lighting used for reading are critical, as far as lighting throughout the rest of the house goes let your feelings be your guide. If you feel comfortable, there's probably adequate light.

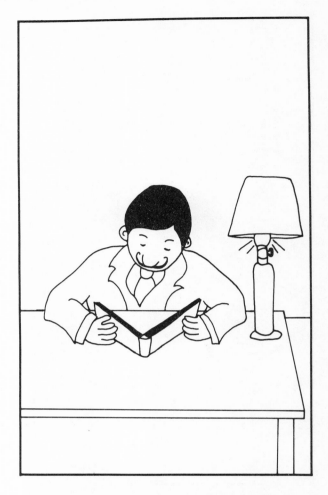

A desk or gooseneck lamp with a 75-watt bulb should be placed about a foot above a book.

You don't have to install old-fashioned overhead lamps in all the rooms, but remember to make use of the lamps that are already there. Probably more of us could *visually* profit (although our pockets wouldn't) by turning on more lights more often. But where close work will be done more specific lighting is important.

A floor lamp which beams the light upward to the ceiling and lets

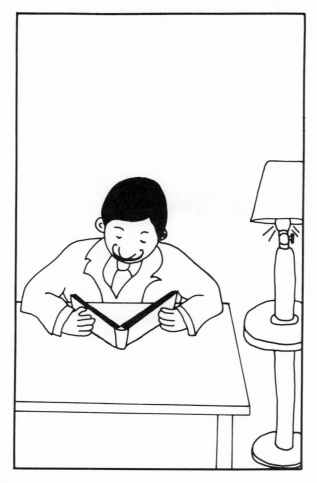

A table lamp with a 100-watt bulb near a desk should be placed off of the left or right shoulder.

it reflect throughout the room can be used instead of overhead lighting. Get one with enough wattage, however; many new lamps are designed for soft, sexy lighting and only hold 60- or 75-watt bulbs. One that takes a three-way bulb up to 250 or 300 watts is acceptable.

Older people, especially, who suffer from the effects of failing vision which accompanies age, notice that reading in dim light is difficult

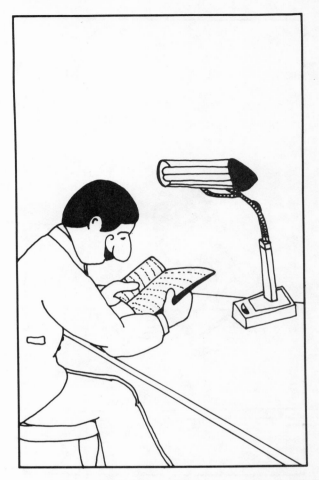

Fluorescent lighting should be provided by full-spectrum fluo-rescent bulbs.

or nearly impossible. Just because you are young and the dimness doesn't bother you does not give you carte blanche to plunge ahead. Turning on a light may save your sight.

The Failure of Fluorescence

While financially strapped school boards and accounting depart-ments of businesses prefer fluorescent lighting because it eats up less power than incandescent, the type of fluorescent tubes that are commonly in use today should carry a warning: *These lights may be harmful to your health—especially if they are the only lighting used during your day.*

Several studies over the last few decades link ordinary fluorescents, which contain only a part of the spectrum of light waves, to a host of general ills far beyond tired and aching eyes—from hyperactivity to cavities. And there is some data suggesting that light may have an effect on the body's glands which may be related to some forms of cancer.

Light, in addition to being necessary for vision, stimulates both the pituitary and pineal glands and possibly other regions of the mid-brain which control the endocrine system and the production of hormones. It is not only the portion of the spectrum which we can see that is important, but also the bands that are present but not visible to the naked eye. The process is not unlike the photosynthesis of plants. Without certain ultraviolet wavelengths human hormone production is altered.

Several researchers working at various medical centers and laboratories throughout the country have found that when any part of the natural sunlight spectrum is blocked from entering the eye for a long period of time, abnormalities may develop. Women living above the Arctic Circle, where the night goes on for three months at a stretch during the winter, are likely to become infertile then because they stop ovulating. When sunlight returns, so does fertility.

Perhaps the most startling relationship disclosed concerning limited-spectrum lighting is the linking to it of some types of cancer. At least a half-dozen animal studies have come up with the same conclusion: reduced-spectrum lighting influences the growth and incidence of some types of cancer. Anything other than the full spectrum appears to change the course of nature.

And when the few reports of remission of terminal cancer in humans are looked at, a connecting link in a number of the cases appears to be getting plenty of natural sunlight. The people decided to spend their last days outdoors in the sun. One such story was reported a dozen years ago in *Time* magazine: the man quit going to his office and started reading in a rocking chair on his back porch and tending roses in his garden. His cancer disappeared.

In a 1959 study with 15 cancer patients at Bellevue Medical Center in New York City, the doctor conducting the research said that while it was difficult to make a definite evaluation, it was her opinion and that of her assistants that 14 of the patients showed no further growth of the cancerous tumors after spending a summer outdoors as much as possible, without wearing sunglasses or prescription lenses.

Subsequently, it was learned that the one patient whose condition deteriorated at the expected rate did not understand the instructions and had continued to wear her prescription lenses when outdoors. The glasses naturally blocked the ultraviolet rays from reaching her eyes.

It appears that not only do we need sunlight on our skin to provide vitamin D from the ultraviolet rays, we also need those invisible rays to reach our eyes, where the nerve fibers in the retina react to stimulate the master glands of the body. (Longwave blacklight ultraviolet rays are the beneficial ones; shortwave ultraviolet, which is filtered from natural sunlight by the atmosphere before reaching us, is so harmful to living tissue that lamps which emit only those bands are used to sterilize implements. Shortwave ultraviolet is also the spectrum emitted from sunlamps, and it has been shown in animal tests that the over-exposure is harmful, possibly causing skin cancer.)

A prominent light researcher, John Ott, tells in his book, *Health & Light,* of a conversation he had with the daughter of the late Dr. Albert Schweitzer:

"Our conversation dwelt mostly on her experiences as assistant to her father at Lambarene, on the west coast of Africa. I asked her about the rate of cancer of the people in that area, and she replied that when her father had first started the hospital, they found no cancer at all, but that now it was a problem. I asked if the people living there had started installing glass windows and electric lights in their otherwise simple surroundings and she said they had not.

"Then I half jokingly asked her if any of the natives wore sunglasses. She looked startled and then told me that the natives paddling their dugout canoes up and down the river in front of the hospital often wore no more than a loin cloth and sunglasses, and indeed, some wore only the sunglasses. She further explained that sunglasses represented a status symbol of civilization and education and had a higher bartering value than beads and other such trinkets. There is, of course, no scientific proof of a correlation between the wearing of sunglasses and cancer, but it does raise an interesting question."

Although we're not all going to look for jobs as oil riggers or farmers—or start paddling canoes under the tropic sun *sans* sunglasses—there is something we can do to help ourselves to better health under indoor and artificial lights: *full-spectrum fluorescents are available and should be installed everywhere possible.*

Incandescent lights, while they lack the full spectrum of natural sunlight, do not appear to cause the same problems as limited fluorescence. Nevertheless, incandescent bulbs are not as good for you as full-spectrum fluorescent lighting. Incandescent bulbs emit little or no ultra-violet and have a graduated continuum which is slanted toward large amounts of red and infrared.

John Ott, retired chairman and executive director of the Environmental Health and Light Research Institute in Fort Lauderdale, developed the full-spectrum fluorescents after spending nearly 40 years observing the effects of lights upon plant growth. His discovery grew out of his work with time-lapse photography for Walt Disney films, which makes flowers appear to grow and blossom right in front of your eyes.

Ott created the full-spectrum by adding the proportionate amount of blacklight to the blend of phosphors currently used in a fluorescent tube. Fluorescents originally were designed to duplicate only the visible wavelengths of natural sunlight; but, as we have pointed out, what you can't see is as important as what you can.

Improved fluorescents are manufactured by several companies: General Electric Chroma 50, Duro-Test Optima, Philips Verd-A-Ray and Vita Lite. They cost a bit more than the limited-spectrum tubes, and the blacklight burns out in approximately a year with normal use, although the tube will still appear to be going strong, making it necessary to replace the fixture before you can see that it needs to be.

Garcy Lighting of Chicago is manufacturing a system which uses regular tubes with a small blacklight tube that can be changed as often as necessary during the normal life of the larger tubes. Called Spectralite, it also eliminates the usual flicker of fluorescence, which has been recognized as a contributing factor to headaches, eyestrain, skin blemishes, fatigue—and has even been known to cause spasms in some epileptics.

The flicker of fluorescence may be using up Vitamin A at a rapid rate, since the rods and cones that transmit color and light are activated by substances that contain a protein and a form of Vitamin A. With each change in lighting these substances either form or dissolve to maintain equilibrium, and the more changes they go through, the more Vitamin A is used up. While each loss is small, it's like taking ladlefuls of soup from a huge pot—you don't notice the difference at first, but eventually the level in the pot gets lower.

As mentioned earlier, we do know that during night driving the off-and-on glare of oncoming headlights consumes Vitamin A rapidly. Although the laboratory research in this area for fluorescents is yet to be done, it may be that the steady but constant stream of short off-and-on flickers gobbles up Vitamin A the same way. As soon as a fluorescent tube has a noticeable flicker, change the tube or check the starter; either may be causing the problem.

Fluorescent tubes have also been found to emit radiation at the terminals, and any type of fluorescent should have shields over the ends of the tubes. In addition, the whole tube should not be enclosed under plastic or glass since *any* covering prevents the full spectrum from coming through. Egg crate designs (with a small grid) cover the tubes but still retain open spaces, thereby reducing glare but letting the ultraviolet and the rest of the spectrum shine down.

It is interesting to note that the salubrious effects of artificial ultra-violets are being put to use in the northern sections of the U.S.S.R., where the sunlight is nil for long stretches of the year. Schoolchildren regularly spend some time in their skivvies being exposed to healthy ultraviolet lighting for a dose of Vitamin D.

Just how bad limited-spectrum lighting is was markedly demonstrated with a group of first graders during the 1973-74 school year in Sarasota, Florida. The four classrooms in the trial were windowless, and thus all lighting was artificial. Two classrooms kept their conventional cool-white fluorescents, and two had full-spectrum lights installed, with shields to reduce radiation.

Under the normal lighting some first graders demonstrated nervous fatigue, irritability, lapses of attention and hyperactivity. Yet when full-spectrum lighting was installed, these same children settled down and paid more attention to their teachers, who reported improved overall classroom performance.

Before the lighting was changed concealed cameras photographed the students fiddling around, leaping from their seats, flailing their arms, and paying little attention.

After two and three months these children were filmed again. Their behavior was entirely different. The children were calmer and more interested in their work.

One little boy stood out in the earlier photographs because of his extreme hyperactivity. After the lighting was changed he became much quieter and was able to sit still long enough to concentrate. His teacher reported that he now was capable of doing independent work, had overcome what appeared to be a severe learning disability and learned how to read in a relatively short time. In those rooms where the lighting was not changed from standard fluorescence, there was no improvement in behavior during this same period of time.

Although this experiment appears to connect conventional fluorescents and possibly some leaking radiation to hyperactivity, it is likely that they are only two of the many causes. In San Francisco, allergist Dr. Ben Feingold has cured some hyperactive children by simply removing all synthetic additives from their diet. His work shows that even a single hot dog can cause a tantrum. What is probable is that some youngsters are more susceptible to certain conditions of modern life than others, and these tendencies are exacerbated by the limited-spectrum lighting.

Cool-white light is probably what is installed in both your office and your children's school. Think about it.

The first graders under full-spectrum lighting also developed significantly fewer cavities than the group who studied under cool-white light. Although the reason for the difference in tooth decay is unclear, these results have been backed up by animal research.

When two groups of hamsters were housed under either full-spectrum fluorescence or lamps lacking ultraviolet and fed the same cavity-producing diet, the group under the full spectrum had fewer cavities than the other group. The difference in lighting produced a difference in the amount and composition of saliva, with the limited-spectrum group having increased potassium and chloride in their saliva.

On the other hand, there has been research indicating that saliva alone bears no relationship to tooth decay. What does appear true, in any event, is that the lighting made a difference. It seems that body chemicals, perhaps hormones, are activated by full-spectrum lighting.

Although all this data has been published in journals over the last several years, it largely has been ignored by the scientific community, and the general public has never heard of it. In this case, ignorance is far from bliss.

How critical adequate lighting is can be inferred from experiments with animals: they developed myopia more quickly under dim conditions than under bright light. The same appears to be true of people. The studies with Eskimos discussed earlier show that a population with almost no myopia went to a full 65 percent in a single generation—the one that learned to read. Although all the research done throughout the world correlates literacy with incidence of myopia, the Eskimos exhibited a greater shift in a few years than other cultures. The offending variable appears to have been lighting. Most Eskimo homes when electrified had a single 40-watt bulb installed in the center of the home, usually a single room approximately 10 feet by 10 feet. Under these dim conditions, the new readers read and read through the long winter night, and quickly became nearsighted.

The lack of sunlight—and its dollop of ultraviolet—also may play a part in what happens to the eye biochemically as it becomes nearsighted. It may be suffering from a lack of Vitamin D and its constant companion, calcium.

It has long been thought that myopia was a biochemical response due to a hormonal imbalance. In researching this book it has occurred to us that since myopes generally read indoors under artificial lights and are not often involved in outdoor activities, they perhaps lack adequate D, which causes a difficulty in absorbing the calcium needed for strong muscles. Some of these muscles control the focus of the eyes. An additional clue is the fact that there has been some success reported in treating myopia with Vitamin D and calcium.

No artificial lighting is as good as natural light. Too many of us get too little of it—maybe only minutes each day running to and from the train to get to the job. If the sun's shining (and for lots of fashion-conscious types, even if it's not) sunglasses are *de rigueur*. Too bad.

Add to that group the 50 percent who wear prescription glasses. Neither type of glasses normally permits the whole range of natural light to come through to the eyes, which, as we have stressed, appears to be important not only for the health of the eyes, but also for our general well-being.

Sitting in the sun in a glassed-in porch or riding in a car doesn't count either. Being outside is necessary. Regular glass blocks ultraviolet. Anyway, you can't get a suntan through the window, a fact which the Kennedys took into account when building their home at Hyannisport. Special quartz windows that let the ultraviolet through were installed in a sunporch. Some hospitals and nursing homes are using a type of plastic window to permit shut-ins to enjoy the sun's benefits. Our suggestion, however, is not to replace your windows but to spend at least a half hour to an hour outdoors daily *without* glasses.

Those used to wearing sunglasses constantly may experience some discomfort without them at first, but this should go away in a few days. You may have become psychologically—if not physiologically—addicted to your shades. If the discomfort doesn't clear up in a few days, seek professional help.

Television

Although the television manufacturers assure us that radiation leakage (X rays) has been reduced to little or none as long as the set is in good working order, you might as well take the precaution of sitting five or six feet away. This is particularly important if your set is color, as they generally emit more radiation. Watch out for younger children especially, as they prefer sitting extremely close to the picture. But don't sit so far away that you have to strain to see the details.

Do not watch television in a darkened room—even if it's the late movie in bed. Looking at a television set is similar to staring at a low wattage light bulb, which is certainly not good for you. By having light all around, the eye strain is somewhat reduced. The lamps should be placed where the light is not reflected on the screen.

And take a break every now and then, just as suggested when doing close work. Children will sometimes sit through hours of Saturday morning cartoons while the parents sleep in. The networks and advertisers of sugar-coated crunchy oats may like it, but the child's mind is intellectually turning off. He may be looking without seeing in the mind's eye of the brain.

This may be related to the fact that a child who watches more than three or four hours a day has been found to have reduced thinking ability, making it much more than merely interesting to speculate about the relationship between the avid TV viewer and the poor or non-reader. We often find that TV addicts look but do not perceive, and frequently exhibit alpha brain waves while reading.

Alpha normally does not even occur when the eyes are open. It is considered to be a nonvisual brain wave. When the eyes open, the brain is supposed to attend to what you are seeing, and alpha normally disappears. It is possible that kids who get zonked on TV fall into alpha during a visual state, and this carries over to other times when they attempt different tasks. Like reading.

Whether overexposure to that black box in the living room is also crippling our bodies as well as our minds is another topic worthy of debate. It may be that low-level X-ray radiation—invisible and insidious—is doing at least as much damage as the diet of crime and violence the networks keep serving up. Although the safety standards have been tightened many times during the past few decades, we are not sure what radiation fall-out—no matter how minute—may be doing to us in the long run. In any event, many experts believe it is not good for us.

When the television sets of a dozen hyperactive children in Sarasota were tested they were found to be giving off low levels of X rays. After the sets were either discarded or repaired, the children, who had been attending a special school because of their learning difficulties, were able to return to regular classes in a matter of months.

In 1963 the "tired child" syndrome was found to correlate to the amount of time spent watching television, and the irritability and fatigue was attributed to the high content of crime and violence of the programs. Similarly, more recent medical reports indicate that air traffic controllers exhibit some of the same symptoms. There is some speculation that this may be related to looking into the tubes of their radar scopes rather than simply the psychological stress of the job. It may be that violence or the threat of a crash is disrupting lives, or it may be the screens' X-ray emissions.

Animal and plant studies are also telling: bean plants and white rats both exhibited abnormal growth when placed directly in front of a turned-on television covered by a sheet of black paper which would block the picture but not the radiation. Yet when the sets were covered with lead shields which block the radiation, growth and behavior returned to normal.

Glasses
While the purpose of this book is to help you help yourself to better vision—and, it is hoped, lead us toward a world where every other person isn't required to wear glasses all the time—there are certain types of lenses which can reduce the stress of near-point focus and help preserve your sight. Optically, *preventive* or *anti-stress* lenses move the object back in space, allowing the focus to be more relaxed. Such lenses have been found to be particularly useful shortly after a youngster learns to read—around seven—and again during other periods of visual stress. The glasses may prevent the myopic syndrome from progressing.

As we have discussed, myopia appears to be directly related to literacy, a result of the long and unrelieved hours of close work which forces the eye into a tight and tense near-point focus. Anti-stress lenses, given at a time when the child first shows signs of becoming nearsighted, make reading less of a strain. The child may still read as much as before, but his eyes are relieved of some of the stress of near-point focus. The lenses are usually not good for anything other than close work, because beyond a distance of two feet the image is fuzzy.

Combined with a program of vision therapy, which sometimes may be done at home, such lenses may make it unnecessary for the individual ever to later need glasses for distance viewing. L.D., for instance, took off her "nearsighted" granny glasses—tinted pink—sometimes during therapy, and conveniently lost them. They haven't been replaced. She describes how and when she uses anti-stress glasses:

Acuity in my left eye was 20/200 when I began vision therapy. The eye had probably weakened from underuse, and from reading in bed with a single lamp off to one side.

The doctor asked if I had trouble concentrating when the subject matter was difficult. Did my mind wander if the material was hard to comprehend? Did I tire easily when reading a medical journal compared to when reading a magazine article? Did I find myself constantly looking up and noticing that maybe I should dust my library shelves? YES. I got anti-stress lenses.

The difference they made as soon as I put them on was remarkable. The words looked easier to understand—and they were! I had never thought that the print of books was dim before, but now it was noticeably more distinct. And although I had never thought that words floated around a bit before, I was now aware that they seemed more stable and easier to comprehend.

I still have the same pair. I wear them whenever I am working at reading or writing, and the concentration demanded is high. I don't consciously think about the fact that they make life easier, I just find myself reaching for them. However, I never think about them when reading lighter material—newspapers, magazines or novels. What I mean is that I don't use them all the time.

My old granny glasses? Don't know what happened to them. Acuity in the bad eye tests at 20/40 on a good day—relaxed, that is—and I don't feel I need them for the movies, as I used to. True, I am aware that clarity in the left eye could be better—I realize it every time I try on somebody else's "nearsighted" glasses—but the difference isn't enough to bother me.

I grew up thinking I had inherited nearsightedness from my father, just the way I acquired his family's voice and my mother's legs. He was intelligent, a reader and a coin collector: he spent hours at near-point focus. And the lighting in the house where he grew up was poor. At 13 he quit school and became a coal miner, thereby getting little exposure to the sun, the source of Vitamin D, whose lack appears to be related to nearsightedness. The condi-

tions could scarcely have been more conducive to myopia. Sure, I inherited many things from my father. I became a reader at an early age. My mother was always after me to shut off the light and go to bed. I got a flashlight and took to reading under the covers.

What happens to the child in school? He complains he can't see the blackboard; the teacher moves him to the front of the room and sends home a note that he should be seen by an eye doctor. He is examined, and indeed, distant images are unclear. No consideration is given to what is causing that. He is prescribed corrective lenses to attempt to make up for the lack of ability on the part of the wearer to see afar. They allow him to see as if he had normal healthy vision without distortion. They make distant images seem more intense and clearer. In effect, the youngster has been handed a crutch. They do not attempt to help the eyes out of the trouble they have gotten into with the hours of reading stress; they merely enforce the abnormal focusing.

Now the child has a pair of glasses which help him see the blackboard from the back row, but what happens when he shifts his focus to the book right in front of him? He probably doesn't take off his glasses then, thereby forcing the eye to get used to seeing at near-point with lenses designed for distance. The eyes become more and more myopic. Next year the glasses prescribed are stronger.

Had the child been given anti-stress lenses, the condition might not have worsened. And he wouldn't end up as an adult who reaches for his glasses the first thing in the morning.

Preventive lenses (sometimes called developmental) are often used in vision therapy, because they allow the exercises to be exaggerated for greater effectiveness. The training lenses, used in therapy sessions under close supervision, may be stronger than those prescribed for outside the office.

The lenses can be used in other ways too. For instance, if one visual skill is far behind the other skills in development, glasses designed for that particular purpose may help the lagging skill to catch up. Sometimes a child will overfocus, which may interfere with eye teaming, or the ability to use both eyes together. This can cause intermittent double vision and loss of place on the page or the sports field. The youngster momentarily loses track of where the ball is and misses the catch. Developmental lenses relax the focus power to a point where it is in line with the eye-teaming ability. By keeping them in balance, eye teaming has a chance to develop and catches up with the other skill.

This may only take a few months, and the glasses are then no longer needed.

Developmental lenses are also useful in enhancing or relaxing a specific visual ability in order to accomplish a specific job, which may be seemingly unrelated to sight. The dentist who is constantly bending over to see critical details—the condition of your pearly whites—is very likely to go on stooping the rest of the time too. If he wears special lenses which appear to bring the floor up toward him, he will automatically push back his head to walk tall.

Because posture both determines and reflects the attitude of the mind, some hyperactive individuals who have trouble concentrating on a point in space benefit from glasses which do the opposite: they push the floor down. In response, the person's posture is focused in and down. His body is ready to attend to the details of nearby space rather than the whole wide world, where his attention flips from one thing to another as fast as they whizz by.

Because any obstruction will block some portion of the spectrum from reaching your eyes, we strongly advise purchasing glasses or contact lenses specially manufactured to allow as much full-spectrum light through as possible. Armorlite is more transparent than glass and regular plastic lenses to visible light and to the long wavelengths found in sunlight. Armorlite lenses are somewhat more costly than regular lenses, but the difference in what they do makes them well worth the extra cost. Full-spectrum contact lenses are manufactured by Wesley-Jessen.

According to Ott, plastic lenses originally were made to let through ultraviolet. At the insistence of the Air Force, which was using the plastic for the windows in their fighter planes, the formula was changed to screen out the ultraviolet so their pilots would be protected from the burning rays at high altitudes. Today, for full-spectrum use, the plastic has to be pulled off the assembly line before the inhibiting factor is included.

Not only should you not wear sunglasses all the time, but the constant wearing of other tinted lenses should also be avoided at all costs. Each color blocks certain light frequencies, i.e., blue lenses stop red waves, rose-colored glasses keep out blue, and so on. In addition to the fact that any interference with the full spectrum is unhealthy, they probably have the effect of subtly altering the way you feel about the world around you. They may make your old blue eyes seem more so, but their psychic costs can be way too high. Just as the colors we wear affect us, so do the tints we see through.

However, there are occasions when tinted lenses are prescribed in order to effect a change visually—but this is done under supervision and for a specific reason.

Because sunglasses should not be worn in normal sunlight but only when the glare is excessive, such as on a beach or ski slope or during exceptionally bright days, photochromatic lenses which automatically change from light to dark in contrast to the available lighting are not a good idea for constant wear. For people who wear glasses constantly they may seem like a great convenience, but they—along with sunglasses worn constantly—take over the adaptation response to light your eyes should be handling by themselves. If you walk around on crutches when you don't need them, your legs become weak, and the same is true of your eyes if you wear sunglasses all the time. Photochromatic lenses, worn constantly, practically guarantee that the wearer will never be without shades when the sun is up.

In time, and after repeated exposure to sunlight, the glasses retain a smoky tinge even at night, putting them into the category of tinted lenses.

In short, wear sunglasses only when you must, and since you want them to reduce glare, get a pair dark enough to do that, dark gray or green, evenly tinted and not gradiently shaded. Your eyes don't tone the scene dark at the top and light at the bottom.

And don't wear your shades at night unless you are escaping from the papparazzi.

Annual Visual Examination

A visual examination—preferably annually—should be as regular as a visit to the dentist. A complete exam should include all aspects of vision: focusing, tracking, peripheral vision, eye/hand coordination, eye teaming—in addition to acuity and disease. A person who has never had a problem with vision may find that as a result of a new job, the needed level of a particular skill suddenly becomes greater and the eyes may be overworked. Vision training—and perhaps a pair of anti-stress lenses—may alleviate the problem and make the job easier. Remember, eye strain causes brain drain.

Tired Eyes

Each day, especially after having used your eyes for long periods of close work, do the following:

Apply hot and cold compresses to your face, brows, lids, cheeks.

Use small towels or washcloths which have been dunked in hot and cold water. The compresses should not be so hot as to burn your eyes.

Apply first one, then the other, ending up with the cold compresses. This helps to open and close the blood vessels in the facial area and reduce swelling from stagnant fluids. Do this for two to three minutes.

Follow this by gently massaging the forehead, lids and upper cheeks with your fingertips. This will tend to maintain normal skin tension.

Sports

Most people do not consider the visual skills involved in sports aside from the most obvious one, acuity, but a number of other basics are frequently needed:

- Eye-movement proficiency allows the individual to attend to the task and know where the object of interest is in the field and where it is going. It gives the person a left-right and up-down focus. If you're going to catch a pass, you'd better know where the ball is headed.
- Eye focus helps in concentrating *on* and *with* the target. It also tells us if the target is coming closer or retreating farther away, and helps us determine how fast a target is moving. Did your opponent hit a drop shot just over the net, or is that a hard drive coming your way?
- Eye teaming is our ability to align both eyes on the target comfortably. This skill acts almost like a range-finder. As the target comes closer, the eyes converge more. As the target moves away, the eyes converge less.
- Peripheral vision and eye/body coordination together give us the ability to move our bodies gracefully through space, maintaining good posture and balance, and orienting ourselves to the activity. A pass receiver must know where he is on the field, where the ball is going, and where those guarding him are. The tennis player has to know where the ball is going and where his opponent is. The skier must not only orient his body to the feel of his skis traversing the slope *right now,* but also anticipate three seconds later when he has to ride that mogul.
- Visualizing the task beforehand gives you a leg up on doing it. Most good athletes will tell you that they do not think of the mechanics of the task when they are actually involved in them. They let their bodies do the work they were trained for, but practice their mechanical skills in their mind by visualizing the task beforehand. They do this

while sitting in an easy chair, while walking to the next chip shot or between serves, but not at the time of the action. Thinking about the mechanics during the swing interferes with coordination and grace.

How helpful this can be was demonstrated a few years ago in an Australian study in which basketball players improved their free shot ability 23 percent just by practicing the shot mentally 20 minutes a day for 20 days.

(For developing some of the above skills, see visual games 1, 8, 10, 16, 21 and 26.)

Nutrition

Food is as critical for the eye as it is for the rest of the body. Because you are not 16, don't feel that you have outgrown the need for good nutrition and vitamins. Especially recommended are increasing the B vitamins; C and its complex form, the bioflavonoids; D, and calcium. While glaucoma and cataracts are major illnesses that take their toll in diminishing sight—if they don't lead eventually to blindness—there is quite a bit of research indicating they may be related to inadequate vitamins, minerals and protein. Chapter 6 deals extensively with nutrition.

Getting Back to the Basics

There are a few simple exercises which should be done by everyone every day. Although some of them seemingly have little or nothing to do with vision, they are designed to relax the body and at least momentarily return it to a state of grace where sight operates the way it was designed to—nice and easy, smooth and relaxed. (The final section of the book contains a section of visual games and activities for adults as well as children to be done from time to time. The following exercises should be done regularly.

Deep Breathing

Stand in a relaxed posture, preferably near an open window (admitting, we hope, clean air). Breathe in through your nose. Keep your mouth closed and your abdomen compressed. Pause for a few seconds. Then let the breath out through your mouth in a smooth manner. Don't keep the breath from coming out; let it escape.

Try to do this for 10 breaths. Stop if you should feel any disturbance or dizzyness.

Body Relaxation

We are not designed to sit still for long periods of time. If we do—and so many of us do—our bodies get tense, and this leads to greater vulnerability for breakdowns in the tissues of our bodies as well as our eyes.

Practice daily some gentle rhythmic movements of your body:

a. While standing in the middle of the room—feet apart about the width of your shoulders—rotate your body to your left and look at an object. Then rotate your body to the right and look at another object. Slowly, smoothly and rhythmically rotate your body from side to side. If you prefer you can do it in time to music.

b. Repeat the above, only this time keep your eyes focused on an object in front of you as you slowly rotate your body from side to side.

c. Repeat procedure (a) with only your head. Rotate your head slowly from side to side, looking at an object at each side as you do this.

d. Repeat the above procedure, except this time focus your eyes on an object in front of you as you rotate your head from side to side.

Continue to do each procedure about 10 times. Stop if you feel uncomfortable or dizzy.

Sunlight Stimulation

To repeat some important points made earlier, try to be outdoors *without* glasses for at least a half hour per day. Look up at the sky. DO NOT FOCUS ON THE SUN. Let the light enter your eyes without being impeded by plastic or glass.

Try to have full-spectrum lights installed at your place of work. These are fluorescents that duplicate natural light. Regular cool-white fluorescents or incandescent lights eliminate some portion of the natural light spectrum and may be deleterious to health.

Circle Fixations

Stand in a relaxed, comfortable manner so that the middle of the target on the next page is lined up with the middle of your nose.

Put on some music with a strong beat.

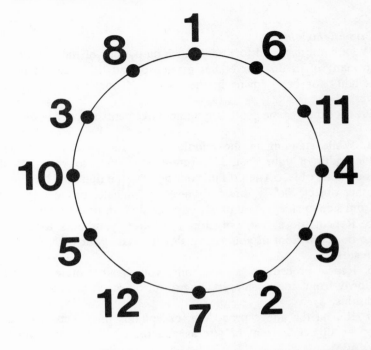

Locate the number 1 with your eyes. At the next beat locate the number 2 out of the corner of your eye—do not move your eye to number 2 at this beat—and on the next beat move your eye to the number 2 in one smooth, accurate movement.

Repeat for all the numbers:

Look at the number on one beat.
Locate the next number on the next beat.
Move your eye to the next number on the third beat.

Focus Shift

Hold a newspaper about 16 inches in front of your eyes. Read one sentence, keeping the letters as clear as you can. Shift your attention to the numbers on a calendar at least 10′ away. Try to see the numbers clearly as quickly as you can.

Move the newspaper toward you by about one inch. Shift your attention to the newspaper again and try to clear the letters as quickly as you can. Read one more sentence. Shift your attention to the calendar again, and then back to the newspaper.

Continue to move the newspaper closer to you, one inch at a time, until you are no longer able to focus on the letters.

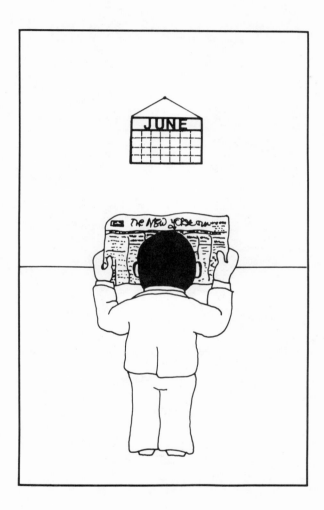

part three

8
Future Sight–Taking Care of Your Child's Eyes

There are two ways to raise a child. We can let him or her grow and develop as chance and disposition dictate, basing parental guidance on intuition and the rules and rituals of the generation.

Or we can provide the child with an intellectually stimulating environment and coax and encourage the youngster to develop intelligence in order to achieve in our world, to be a chemist or a veterinarian, a teacher or a newspaper reporter. But we may do that at the expense of the child's healthy vision.

When a child walks through school doors for the first time, he enters the adult visual world where he will be assaulted with a complex network of tiny details—letters and numbers—through which he is expected to learn. It starts with the alphabet and ends up with cell biology a decade or two later.

On the first day of school his life drastically alters from one of days of fun and games to long periods of sitting still and concentrating. Eye/hand coordination is largely replaced with eye/brain cooperation.

The educational system seems designed to ruin his sight by requiring him to attend to details hour after hour, and the result can be seen in the fact that half the population wears glasses. To give a pair of young eyes a fighting chance against the visual requirements of life today, they should at least start out with healthy vision, normal for their age. This requires that parents help a child learn how to see properly. We hold onto a toddler when he takes his first shaky steps as he learns to walk; his eyes need a different kind of help. Because we can't see a pair of eyes grow up and learn doesn't mean that they don't.

The amount of research today about how sight grows and vision develops has accumulated to the point where we can no longer be unaware of what's going on in a child's eyes and blithely assume that everything will turn out for the best.

How a child grows and learns and is able to use his eyes, his windows on the world, will largely determine the abilities he will have to carry him on through life. Although all the skills—motor, sensory and mental—play their individual part in a whole person, the visual abilities are primarily responsible for coordinating the system. For twentieth-century man and woman, vision is especially critical, since so much of the information we gain about the world comes to us through our eyes. In our literate culture we ask our eyes to take on a job for which evolution has not yet prepared them: close concentration hour after hour, paying attention to details, reading words, adding or subtracting numbers or punching them out on a calculator.

The message of the times is: achieve in this manner or fall by the wayside. In their effort to achieve, some develop visual problems; others are held back because of them.

But there is a great deal a parent can do to help a child develop healthy vision and adult perception. Following is a compendium of activities from birth to six years.

Birth to Two Months

Although an infant's eyes look pretty much like an adult's, his vision is undeveloped. He can see light and pattern at birth, but anything beyond eight inches is a blur. That's close enough for important things, however, like mama's face when she holds him.

• An infant needs to have bright spots and shadows in his environment in order to begin developing his visual abilities, so keep a dim light on in the nursery at night. This provides something to look at whenever he awakens and gives him the opportunity to learn how to point his eyes.

• Don't push the crib up against one wall and leave it there. Change its position frequently, allowing him to respond to light coming from different directions. This also gives him the chance to use both eyes rather than only the one facing away from the wall. If you can't move the crib around, change the child's position each time you place him back in his crib. Remember, at his age, he can't move his head from side to side by himself. Move the furniture or him instead. Cribs or bassinets with solid sides are poor choices for his bed for he can not see through them.

• Hold the infant on opposite sides during meal time, as a mother does naturally if she is breast feeding. This allows for equal use of both eyes. Likewise, vary the side from which his diaper is changed.

• By the time the child is five or six weeks old he is aware of different patterns of light and is ready to have his visual environment enriched. Hang a mobile within a foot of his eyes. Don't go wild with gizmoes which wiggle, and printed sheets, however, because overkill of visuals results in an infant shutting off some of it, which slows development. Infants with a moderate number of things to look at progress the most rapidly. Small doses of color and sound go a long way.

• Talk to him from different areas of the room. This gives him a moving target to watch and follow, allowing him to associate distance and direction with both sight and hearing.

• Let your child spend some of his waking time in rooms other than the nursery, providing him with more bright areas and objects to watch while learning to control his eye movements.

• Along with things to watch, a child needs to start moving his head around as soon as possible. This can be encouraged by placing him on his stomach for five or 10 minutes at a time—unless, of course, he informs you he doesn't like it. He'll let you know right quick.

Two to Four Months

Somewhere around 14 weeks both eyes converge, which starts to give an infant better depth perception. While before he saw only a two-dimensional, flat picture of a face, now he prefers the texture and depth of a real face, or a sculpted one.

As this big new world becomes familiar, we see the beginnings of memory, for he will pay more attention to new objects than ones he's used to, which should make the manufacturers of baby rattles happy. Now he starts swiping at objects. He's learning that he can reach out with his arm and actually touch that purple and pink hippopotamus mama is holding. He can touch mama's nose, too.

Although an eye may turn in or out now and then, it shouldn't always be in the same direction nor for hours at a time. If this occurs, the child should be examined by a vision therapist immediately. The longer the aberration is allowed to remain, the harder it will be to make it go away.

• Move the mobiles over the center of the child's body. Now that he can turn his head, toys and such objects should not always be on one side.

• Put the child in a sturdy, stable child's seat, allowing him to watch his mother or father during the day. The seat should be put where it won't easily tip over, or, if it does, where the infant won't fall far.

• During these months, posture begins to change, and the baby's head is no longer turned to one side but held more often in the middle. On his stomach, he will attempt to raise his chest to look around. Let him try this out by putting him on his stomach frequently.

• As soon as possible, the infant should be given plenty of space to roam around in, wearing as few clothes as possible, since all garments restrict movement to some degree. Letting a baby explore the world of his blanket on the floor without diapers may be chancy, but Junior will love it—and learn. Make sure there is no draft near the floor. Diapers aren't the worst things that a child endures, but being hauled around wrapped up tightly limits his opportunity to practice his motor skills and coordinate them with what he sees.

• Give him a non-breakable mirror without sharp edges. The child enjoys communicating with his new friend.

• Toys and other things to reach for should still be within eight inches, the distance he can focus. They should be easy to grasp, and not pull toys. That's much too complicated for right now.

Four to Six Months

The child now should be able to turn himself from one side to the other, and his use of arms and legs is picking up. And by this time, what the eye sees, the brain can direct the hand to grab. You may think it's only noise when he bangs a rattle on his high chair, but it's a symphony to him, composed, directed and written all by him. He is learning about coordination.

He should now be able to turn his eyes, his head, his whole body to attend to a sound. He is learning about motor skills. Exploring textures and shapes with his fingers will be highly entertaining to him. He's learning about touch, and how something that feels bumpy *looks;* that blue is not necessarily smooth, even though his rattle is. By this time he should have control of his eyes so there is no eye drifting.

• Make sure the child can see out of the crib on both sides and has interesting things to look at. Place him on a blanket on the floor so he can watch the action in the room. All too often a child is treated like an alien, shut off from the rest of the family in his room. No matter how it's decorated, it isn't as interesting as being a part of the group and seeing what the big folks do.

- Get a strong crib gym with a bar and lots of gadgets he can hold onto and pull.
- Put toys in the crib that move or make music when pulled.
- Hang objects across the crib to foster eye and foot coordination. He will be very interested in kicking up his heels. After all, he just found out he can do that.
- Give him objects of all textures and shapes. He'll try them out with his fingers before they go into the mouth.
- Play "patty cake," manipulating his hands rhythmically and saying the words as you do.
- Tie bells on his booties—he'll enjoy kicking his feet to see and hear the new attraction down there.
- Before he begins to crawl, he could use a little help from a small but hard bolster, placed under his abdomen, which allows him to roll over it. This will help get him moving through space.

At six months the child should have a complete visual examination to make sure that everything is chugging along the way it's supposed to, because a roadblock at such a young and malleable age often can easily be set aside before it interferes with learning or causes an emotional scar. A vision examination every six months by a behavioral optometrist should be as ordinary as a visit to the pediatrician until the child is five, when most of the visual apparatus has developed. An annual examination ordinarily will suffice after that.

One little boy was examined at six months because his mother was aware that he should be grabbing for objects at that age but wasn't. His eyes did not seem to pinpoint their focus, which would help him locate objects and guide his hands. He had a dull, glazed look. The examination found that indeed he was not focusing and couldn't see well enough to reach out with any accuracy. The child was given developmental lenses to wear which boosted his focusing ability.

Within a day he started grabbing and throwing things on the floor. He throws it down, you pick it up; he throws it down, you pick it up; he throws it down—it's a fun game for him. And it's how he begins learning about space.

By the end of the week he reached up and took off his glasses. He didn't need them anymore. They had put his eyes back on the right track, and he now was used to seeing in a healthy manner, rather than repeating a bad visual habit and making it a part of his behavioral repertoire.

During an examination, an infant won't be expected to read letters on a chart or to put up calmly with a procedure he doesn't understand, but there are ways of making it all a jolly game. Do the child's eyes follow a target—say a toy—as it's moved past his eyes? Does he follow it smoothly from one side to the other? Does he focus clearly enough to see that tiny jelly bean placed in front of him? Does he grab for it and put it in his mouth? Is his body coordination developing in line with his visual skills, and at the normal rate? Does he make eye contact? Or does he seem not to see you?

To measure whether or not the eye is coming to focus where it is supposed to, a retinoscope is used, the same instrument that is used to shine a light in an adult's eyes. The beam bounces off the back of the eye, and where it comes to a focus outside is the basis for determining the focal length of the eye, which indicates the optical distortion if it's off the norm.

Many examiners use drops to "still" the eye, but the measurement under medication is frequently different from the one obtained without drugs. Infants will often show a higher amount of farsightedness than is usual. If glasses are prescribed for this amount, which may well be artificially created by the drops, the child's eyes may eventually conform to the lenses. The following year a stronger prescription may well be needed. Instead of alleviating a problem, the glasses actually caused one.

The child's final prescription should be determined by many factors: do other symptoms confirm the measurement with the drops? What is the measurement under normal—drug-free—conditions? Is this finding typical for his age? Too many examiners believe that medication must be used to force total relaxation of the child's eyes in order to obtain an accurate measurement.

Totally relaxed eyes—during sleep—wander up and out, except while dreaming, when they move around as if watching an inner videotape. Yet no one suggests that those up and out eyes are indicative of what they should be like in a waking, normal state. This is not to say there are not times when the drops are useful, such as when checking for disease or examining an unusually hyperactive child.

Six to Eight Months

The child is gaining control of all of his parts—arms, legs, neck, head. What he cannot do yet is get his torso moving through space upright, but he will begin to crawl and should be allowed to as freely as possible. Naturally, you can't turn a whole house into a nursery without sharp edges, but the infant should not be confined to a playpen for hours on end. He needs to get around to practice using both sides of his body, against the time when he is ready to explore his environment. But he won't be interested in venturing out beyond the house or apartment yet, and he is beginning to be afraid of strangers. This is a time of forming an enduring attachment to the primary care-giver, usually mom. And by the end of this period he'll probably be able to say her name: *mama.*

He will be examining time and space relationships—what happens when I do this? This means banging toys, dropping them, turning lights on and off, and opening and closing doors will be fascinating to the youngster. It will pass.

Now he can see an object one-eighth of an inch in diameter held at arm's length—his, not yours. He should be able to use each eye easily, and show no greater discomfort if you cover one eye or the other. Both eyes should focus equally.

The schedule of growth outlined here is not rigid, and individual differences will have one child doing something ahead of the norm but lagging behind in another skill. However, the deviation should not be more than a few months behind what is expected, and this includes all aspects of a child's development: motor skills, movement, visual ability, perception and language. Out of these aptitudes interpersonal relationships and intelligence will grow, based on what nature put there and the type of nurturing it receives from the care-givers—Mom and Pop and Sister Sue.

• Provide toys that have simple mechanisms such as a jack-in-the-box or a door which opens or a switch which flicks.

• Play hide-and-seek games. Put a ball under a blanket or chair and ask him where it is. He will be delighted with his perception and memory.

• Talk concretely in the here and now about what he is doing. Speak in short sentences, but not saccharine baby talk. Use auxiliary words such as *will, may, could,* and address him in questions when they are called for. Studies indicate that the child's language will be more sophisticated if you do, but don't expect miracles. (And when he does start talking, somewhere around 12 months, it's best not to correct him right away. You may wind up doing it too much, and he'll be getting only negative feedback for his valiant efforts. The important thing is communication, not grammar.)

• Roll a ball back and forth to him. Have him sit so that the ball will roll between his legs. Tennis is an adult version of this eye-tracking exercise.

• Provide stacking toys, stuffed animals, and objects with details. He's ready to look at the finer points of larger objects.

Eight to 14 Months

During the next six months, Junior seems to really grow up. Now that he's gotten used to the world outside the womb, he's learning how to manipulate it, learning the skills with which we control our environment: walking, talking, taking things apart and putting them back together.

He will begin to use two eyes to judge distance, and throw objects with precision. He is conquering the battle with gravity now. He's climbing, standing and cruising while holding onto furniture or walls. At 12 to 15 months he's walking, and then running. His thumbs and fingers are coordinated so that he will be able to release things when he wants to, not just when the muscles relax, which is what happened before. He understands as well as an adult that there are things he must learn how to do well, and will practice and practice until he gets them right. Junior might decide that it is time to learn how to take a step up and a step down. He will do it over and over again, never getting bored, until he is satisfied he can do it well.

• When you talk to him, label objects in his environment: the toaster, the puppy, the furry mittens for cold days. Let him know what he is doing—walking, running, jumping. Vocabulary is learned, and a mother or father who sits there and goes through picture books pointing out and labeling—along with teaching him what is in his own environment—is nourishing the verbal skills.

• Provide small objects to handle, such as spoons, large pegs and dowels. This will lead to the handling of crayons and pencils, the tools he will use to start scribbling with before he writes.

• Give him objects he can roll, especially ones which vary their movement, such as footballs, Silly Putty, and crazy bounce balls.

• Provide toys he can take apart and put back together. Nothing too complicated—he's not ready for mechanisms which require each hand to have a separate activity.

• Provide stiff cardboard books. He will especially like ones with pop-ups, moving parts, or pages you scratch and sniff. Just as he loves to open and close doors, he'll enjoy turning pages back and forth.

• Provide him plenty of opportunity for water play. Although the water won't always stay in the tub or sink, he'll have a great time splashing and listening to how it sounds, feeling how it feels. And perhaps later he won't be afraid to stick his head in when it's time to learn to swim.

During the entire first year and a half, the child is learning how to transform basic reflexes into coordinated activities involving the use of the different senses. Bit by bit he learns that he can exercise control over his environment by making things happen. The more success he has in his little world, the more likely he is going to believe that he has control over his life when he grows up. Which is why it is important not to push a child into activities until he is ready for them. It is better to be successful in a small project than to fail at a grand one.

As adults we tend to follow the path of least resistance. We repeat those activities which are accomplished easily, which bring us joy and fulfillment; we avoid those we are unable to complete and which continually remain beyond our grasp. Frustration turns into anxiety, which turns into the stresses that chip away at the ego and wear out the body. Childhood is a time to get used to the feeling of success.

14 Months to Two Years

The child should have his depth perception fairly well developed and his body coordinated at this stage, so that walking, going up and down steps on all fours, jumping and running are accomplished easily. Eye/hand coordination is fairly smooth. Things go where he puts them.

He is beginning to feel comfortable with his own abilities to get around and take care of himself and is interested in that great big unfamiliar world outside the front door. Although still cautious about strangers, he attempts to make contact with other children his age.

• Provide objects and games which have unusual happenings, such as Silly Putty, kaleidoscopes, finger paints.

• Ask him to think about the consequences of what he is doing. Not in the philosophical realm—just ask him to think about familiar, everyday actions. If you tip the glass, what will happen? If you turn the faucet, what will happen?

• He's ready to conceptualize in the abstract and begins to understand that the big red dog is the same as the little spotted puppy is the same as the great big fluffy one with hair over his eyes. Show him houses that are big, houses that are small. Different kinds of fish and flowers.

• Ask him to carry out complicated activities, like "find the round toy in the den under the red chair." For him, it's a big job—and he'll be overjoyed when he does it right. He knows he's growing up. He couldn't do that two months ago.

Two to Three Years
• He's able to identify parts of his body and other spaces and sizes. He begins to understand that a word like *big* is relative. There are big trees and big balls. He will begin to speak in sentences and enjoy scribbling with paper and crayons, and by the time he's three, he'll end up drawing circles. He's more interested in looking and listening, when before he wanted to look and do. He can conjure up a picture in his mind's eye. Tell him a story and he'll see it happen in his head.

Between two-and-a-half and three the child goes through a period which appears to be a setback. Where before he was coordinated, now he stumbles or misses as he reaches for something. And while this is occurring, he is temporarily vulnerable; it is at this time that many a child's eyes will cross. If this happens the child should be seen immediately by a vision therapist, for the eye can usually be straightened. If caught early enough, the behavioral complications which may result if it is left untreated will not become imbedded in his personality. He is not going to "grow out of it" by himself.

All too often that's the advice that's heard. Yet, if a child had a broken leg, it would be set in a plaster cast; we would hardly listen to the prognosis of a pediatrician who said that the bone would heal itself. True, a crossed eye might *appear* to go away by itself, but it might not. It might get stuck and stay for the full course, just the way a broken bone—without a little help from plaster—will probably mend with a bend. And even if the eye appears to uncross and look sharp and stay straight, it is likely that the inner problem which caused the outer defect is still there, displaced for the time being, which could be as long as a lifetime.

• The "terrible twos" are the time to give the child toys he can manipulate: blocks, crayons, fingerpaints, clay and Play Doh. He's ready to use these implements to create toys and designs out of his imagination. Toys that have parts that snap off and on to make different objects are better than toys that do just one thing.
• Provide plenty of old clothes for costumes. This gives the child a chance to try role-playing and to imagine what it would be like to be

somebody else. Or something else—a walrus or a giraffe. If you don't have an old trunk in the attic full of old clothes, give him family castoffs. Even a selection of hats will be fun for him.

• Make the child aware of good visual habits at this age. He should have adequate light for play and drawing. Some children will start reading, or at least looking at picture books. Proper posture and lighting should be stressed, especially with those who are obviously going to become bookworms. Make sure the visual activity isn't done in an area surrounded by deep shadows.

• This is the time to discourage the child from sitting hour after hour reading. Have him take frequent breaks and move around, and look up every 20 minutes and focus on something in the distance for at least a minute. Habits like this are not formed overnight, which is why adults reading this book who may have the best intentions of following our suggestions will often have difficulty remembering to do them.

Three to Five Years

The child should have a balance of activities. He should not be sedentary all the time, nor should he always be outdoors running and jumping. He'll have too much trouble when school starts. But the little girl who learned how to read and doesn't want to do anything else—or the youngster who has four hours of "favorite" television shows daily— needs to be encouraged to use the whole body and get it moving through space and exercising large muscles. Make acrobatics a game, or dance daily with the child to his favorite songs on the radio. Help these children get in tune with their bodies so they can grow up to be flexible adults with more than one way of expressing themselves.

The child should also start learning how to tone down excitement and relax, because this ability will be important not only when he starts school but later in life. Like so many other things, the earlier one learns how to relax, the less tense the adult will be. The best way to reduce stress is to prevent it. A practice used in yoga can be helpful, and it will seem like a new game to the child:

Have the child lie down on the bed or the floor and concentrate on tightening up various parts of the body, and then relaxing them, one at a time. You might say something like "Tighten up your left leg . . . tighter . . . tighter . . . tighter . . . lift it off the floor a few inches . . . hold your breath . . . and then let it go *mush*." Now on to the right leg, and up the body. This is especially good if the child shows any signs of becoming hyperactive. You want to teach the child to let go the right way, not have an explosion every now and then.

• Teach the child to use his body in as many different ways as possible. How can you move your eyes? Can you look at your nose? Can you look off to the sides? Can you roll your eyes around? Can you wiggle your toes? Your ears? Can you separate your toes? If a child does not have control over his body, his limitations will control him.

• Ask the child to scrunch up his body and make it as small as possible. Then make it as big as possible—stretch it way, way out.

• Ask him to walk by an object as closely as he can without touching it. Have several children walk around each other in circles, coming closer and closer, in smaller and smaller circles, without touching.

• Play the subway game. Have children stand as closely together as possible—without pushing, naturally.

• To help the child understand how big he is, have him lie down on a big piece of wrapping paper, and draw his outline so he can see what his size looks like. Mark his height on the inside of a door and date it. Do it a month later. A child finds all of these activities fascinating because they are about himself. And he's young enough to feel that doing something physical has the same value as quietly reading, or other such intellectual activities. If he's well grounded and sure of his body as a youngster he will be less prone to distorting his body as a way of compensating for the pressures of the school years, and after. A healthy body and a healthy mind may help maintain healthy vision.

• To foster good balance, build a simple walking rail, consisting of two two-by-fours laid side to side and elevated at each end by a book. Ask the child to walk across the board with his arms out: forward, backward, sideways to the middle, and then go . . . backward. Now do it while holding something in one hand. You want to teach the child to walk with balance and grace. Will he think this is boring? Not at all—until he's mastered it, and then he'll enjoy showing off his proficiency. When he's able, let him walk on one two-by-four. Some children will even start skiing in these early years. There is a pair of identical twins in Aspen who can't remember a time when they didn't know how to ski.

Children will probably do some of these balance activities by themselves when they are outdoors cruising around. Think of all the times you walked all the way home from school on the curb, just to prove to yourself that you could do it without losing your balance. Or you walked along a ledge—the narrower the better, the higher the scarier. The coordination and balance learned now will not only make simple movement easier, but will give the child better control of his body when he takes up sports and makes that first run to home base or that first downhill run.

Coordination also allows the child to sit with more comfort and grace, so that he does not distort his body when he starts school. As we have discussed elsewhere, posture is important so that vision is not distorted. And if a child is uncomfortable, he'll gnash his teeth and could end up with a bad bite. Or he'll jump around because sitting doesn't feel good.

• Eye movement skills can be practiced, too. Take a piece of paper and write three figures (letters, numbers or small circles and squares) at the top: one at the left, one in the middle, one at the right. Ask the child to look at the left one, then move to the center, and then to the right. You can have him count as he looks. When he gets better at looking from one to the other, increase the number of figures. His eyes look, stop and move on. If he is looking accurately he will count accurately, but to be sure, watch his eyes as they move. Emphasize looking from left to right, because this will help him get used to the way he will read in our culture. As his eyes get more adept at looking from one figure to another, add a second and third row.

• To introduce form and shape and touch, have a *feelie box*. Put objects he recognizes into a bag or box, ask him not to look while he reaches in and identifies what he touches. Have him pull it out to see if he is right.

• Another way to get him used to form is to have him match objects. Put an array of objects—a red potholder, a yellow crayon, a blue pencil, a brown pencil—in front of you and the same types of things in front of him. Hold up one object and ask him to pick up its counterpart. Once the child can do this, move on to smaller and smaller details—a truck with one wheel missing, a hat with feathers, a hat with a flower.

• Have him try visual games 1, 2, 8, 10, 12, 14, 21.

As your child is growing up, you want to make sure that he is developing good visual-body coordination skills. The following questions may give you a clue if he's running into trouble: Is he clumsy? Does he frequently trip or fall over objects, or bump into them? Does he have good eye/hand coordination for zipping zippers, tieing shoelaces, using crayons? Does he have a short attention span for visual activities such as reading, coloring or drawing? Does he squint? Does he get knocked over more than his friends when he plays soccer? Does he thrust his head forward to look at distant objects? Does he complain of headaches, dizziness or an upset stomach after spending time on a visual task? Does he tilt his head off to one side? Does he hold a book close to his eyes?

All are indications that something is amiss, and the trouble could be visual. Help him get rid of the problem before it becomes big trouble.

Dr. Arnold Gesell's extensive studies of child development led him to say: "Visual defects and deviations express themselves not so much in failures of acuity as in discoordinations, various forms of awkwardness, faulty timing and hesitations. . . . Vision is so completely identified with the whole child that we cannot understand the phenomenon without investigating the whole child."

9
Visual Games

1. Room Fixations

Purpose: To be able to expand your peripheral vision and to be able to shift your vision accurately to any area within your vision.

Materials: None

Procedure: Sit comfortably in a room with many objects to look at, placed at different distances from you. This can also be done while sitting in the park, etc.

Look at an object. At the same time, become aware of all the other objects within the periphery of your vision.

Mentally select another object to attend to. Watch that object with your peripheral vision, while you continue to look at the original object, person, etc.

When you are ready to shift your gaze, do so in a smooth, accurate movement.

As you look at the new object, try to keep the original object, as well as the rest of your field of view, within your peripheral vision.

Repeat this procedure with other objects.

Goals: Try to increase the volume of your peripheral awareness. Learn to locate objects accurately in your periphery and how to shift your gaze to them whenever you want.

2. Pegboard Fixations

Purpose: To locate objects accurately in your periphery and to move your eyes accurately from one to the other in a sequence similar to reading.

Materials: Pegboard (approximately 5 by 5 inches), pegs

Procedure: Place three pegs in the top row of the board: one at the left, one in the middle, and one at the right end. Repeat this line-up in each of the first four rows. Hold the pegboard at arm's length.

During this entire exercise, try to see all the other pegs with your peripheral vision.

First, look at the top left peg. Shift your gaze to the top center peg.

Next shift your gaze to the top right peg.

Shift your gaze to the first peg on the second row. Then to the second and the third pegs on the second row.

Continue with the third and fourth rows as before, until you have looked at each peg by shifting your eyes smoothly and accurately from peg to peg.

As your skill in accurate fixation improves, add more pegs per line and more lines of pegs.

When this exercise is used with children, ask the child to count the pegs. This tends to help the child make more accurate eye stops.

Goal: Smooth accurate eye stops in a left to right direction as in reading.

3. Chalkboard Fixations

Purpose: To develop the ability to locate accurately objects in space with your peripheral vision.

Materials: 3 by 2 foot chalkboard or large piece of construction paper, the letters of the alphabet, written randomly on the surface of the

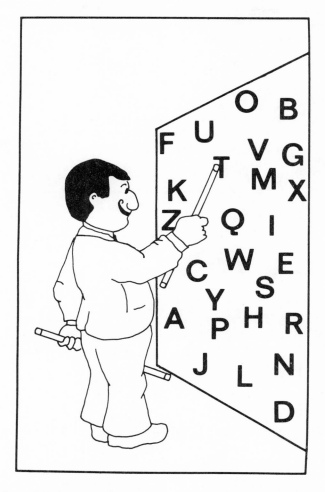

chalkboard, a dowel stick or ruler, approximately three feet long

Procedure: Stand in a relaxed, comfortable position, approximately three feet from the board.

Point to each of the letters of the alphabet with your pointer while alternating hands. Try not to move your body or your head.

To make the exercise more interesting, try to spell words, moving each hand in time to a metronome (at 60 beats per minute) or a good rhythm record.

Goals: To keep all the letters in view at one time. To be able to alternate your hands without confusion.

4. Baseball Fixations

Purpose: To develop the ability to locate objects with your side vision and move your eye accurately from one to the other.

Materials: Six picture baseball, football or movie star cards, approximately 2 by 3 inches

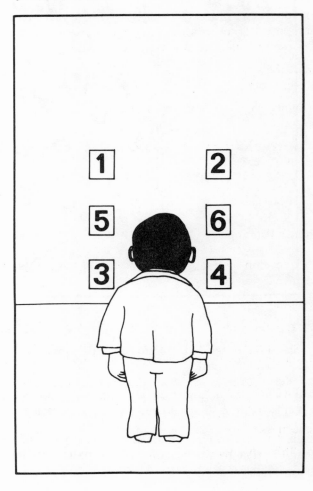

Procedure: Place the cards on the wall in two columns approximately three feet apart. Place them so that the middle two are at eye level. The top two and the bottom two should be three feet above and three feet below the middle cards. Stand in a relaxed, comfortable manner about six feet from the wall so that the middle of your body is lined up with the middle of the pattern.

Look at the picture on the top left. In a smooth, rhythmical manner, shift your eye from the top left to the top right, then to the bottom left, then to the bottom right, then the middle left to middle right and finally return to the top left.

When you can do this easily without having to make any corrective eye movements, have someone call out the picture you are to look at. Try not to anticipate any movements.

Goals: The ability to locate objects accurately out of the corner of your eye.

The ability to move your eyes smoothly and accurately in all directions.

The ability to locate an object peripherally without making any anticipatory movement.

5. Thumb Fixations

Purpose: To develop the ability to move your eyes smoothly from one place in space to another.

Materials: None

Procedure: Extend your arms in front of you, approximately your shoulders' width apart. Make a fist with your thumbs pointing into the air. You should be able to see the fingernail on each thumb.

Direct your eyes to your left thumb. Try to see it clearly. Out of the corners of your eyes be aware of your other thumb. Now shift your eyes to your right thumb. Try to make the shift as smoothly and effortlessly as you can.

Repeat this procedure three or four times. When you have accomplished this, repeat the procedure with:

a) your thumbs held at the midline of your body, one 12 inches above eye level the other 12 inches below eye level. Shift your eyes from top thumb to bottom thumb, back to top thumb, etc. Your eyes should make straight vertical movements. Do this three or four times.

b) position your arms so that they are again a shoulder's width apart, but with the left one above eye level and the right one below eye level. Make straight diagonal movements. Do this three or four times.

c) repeat above procedure, this time with the right hand higher than the left.

Goals: Smooth, easy eye movements from one thumb to the other without extra movements.

Peripheral awareness of the other thumb and, if possible, the rest of the room, at all times.

6. Follow the Imaginary Bug

Purpose: To develop the ability to visualize and then use this skill to control your eye movements.

Materials: None

Procedure: Stand in a relaxed, comfortable manner about eight feet in front of a wall. Picture an imaginary bug or other object on the left top corner of the wall.

Imagine that the bug is moving slowly across the wall to the right. Your eyes should follow it in a slow, smooth, continuous movement. Try to feel the movement of your eyes. If you have difficulty moving your eyes smoothly, point your finger at the bug, but do not look at your finger. The movement of your hand following the bug will help to smooth out the eye movement. When you can move your eyes smoothly using your hand, continue with the exercise with your eyes only.

Continue to follow the bug across to the right, then down the wall, then across the floor to the left, and finally up the wall to the starting point.

Remember: Move only your eyes, not your head or body.

Goal: Smooth, easy, continuous eye movements while maintaining an imaginary bug in the mind's eye.

7. Thumb Pursuits

Purpose: To have your hand teach your eye where you are looking.

Materials: None

Procedure: Extend your hand at arm's length directly in front of your nose.

Make a fist, excluding your thumb. Point your thumb to the ceiling, so that you can view the thumbnail.

Visually concentrate on your thumbnail. Move your hand in the following directions:

| *side to side* | *up and down* | *diagonally* | *circularly* |

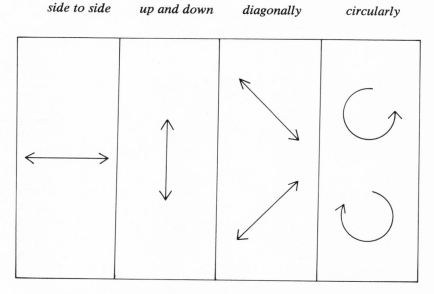

Move your hand smoothly, trying to follow just as smoothly with your eyes.

Try not to move your body or head.

Keep your body relaxed.

When you can do this part of the procedure, repeat it with your eyes closed, following your thumb by visualizing where it is in your mind's eye and by being aware of where it feels like your hand is.

Every so often, open your eyes to check that you're aiming accurately. When you open your eyes they should be looking at your thumbnail.

Try this exercise using each hand.

Goals: Smooth, accurate eye tracking.

Ability to visualize movement.

8. Eye Tracking

Purpose: To develop the ability to move your eyes smoothly and effortlessly.

Materials: A small flashlight (or a popsicle stick with a small target pasted on it)

Procedure: Cover one eye, and hold the flashlight directly in front of the other. You can have someone help you by holding the flashlight.

Move the flashlight slowly and smoothly in the following directions:

| *side to side* | *up and down* | *diagonally* | *circularly* |

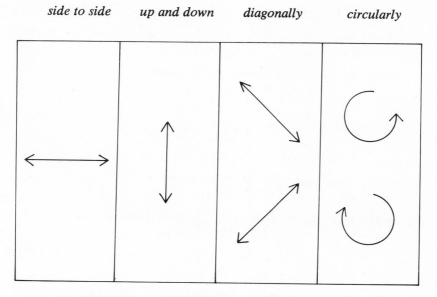

Try to follow the flashlight with your eye in as smooth a fashion as you can while the light is moved.

Try to do this without strain or head or body movements.

Goal: Free and easy eye tracking, with no head or body movements.

9. Focusing Stimulation

Purpose: To help increase your ability to see clearly at the reading distance.

Materials: Newspaper

Procedure: Hold the newspaper approximately 16 inches in front of your eyes. Read the smallest words you can.

Slowly move the newspaper closer to your face until the words blur.

At this point, slowly move the newspaper away from you until the words are *just* readable.

Repeat the exercise.

At the end of the exercise make sure you can relax and see distant objects clearly.

Goal: Maintenance of clear vision at a closer and closer distance.

10. Focusing Pursuits

Purpose: To maintain an accurate focus on a moving target.

Materials: Newspaper type letters pasted on a small stick (A tongue depressor is ideal.)

Procedure: Hold the letter-stick 16 inches in front of your eyes with the letters facing you (see diagram on next page).

Slowly move the stick in a circle, first closer to you and then farther away.

Try to maintain clear vision throughout the entire movement, which should be clockwise first, then counterclockwise.

If you can continually maintain clear vision, slowly increase the size of the circle, especially in the movement toward you.

Repeat the exercise by circling down toward you, then up and away from you.

Goal: Smooth, easy shifting of your focus.

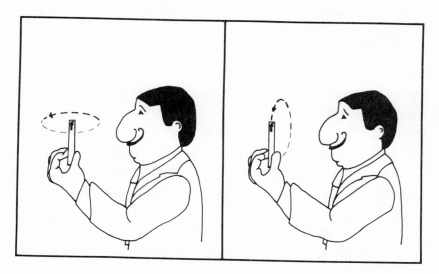

11. The Image Maze

Purpose: To develop eye-hand coordination.

Materials: A 12-inch square peg board, 20 pegs, a small flashlight, sheet of Plexiglas (about 4 by 8 inches)

Procedure: Make a maze on the peg board with the pegs.

Place the pegboard on a table so that you can see the maze.

Stand the Plexiglas sheet upright between you and the maze.

Turn the flashlight on and note the image of the flashlight bulb in the Plexiglas. (You may have to turn all other room lights out for this exercise).

As you move the flashlight, you will see its image move in the Plexiglas as if it were moving in space behind the Plexiglas.

Trace the maze with the light image, by carefully moving the flashlight.

Goal: Good two-eye teaming in coordination with your hands.

12. Balance Ball

Purpose: To develop eye-hand (wrist) coordination.

Materials: Rubber ball, tube from inside roll of paper towels, books of various sizes

Procedure: Hold the tube vertically with the ball balanced on top.

Walk around balancing the ball while holding the tube first with both hands, then either hand, then alternate hands.

Do this while looking at the ball or while looking elsewhere.

As you improve, try to balance the ball (without the tube) on a large book, then on successively smaller books.

Goal: Increased coordination of vision, balance and wrist.

13. Ball Bunt

Purpose: To develop eye-hand coordination and space-time perception.

Materials: Ball suspended from the ceiling; paper towel roll tube

Procedure: Face the ball with hands holding each end of tube at chest level. The palms of both hands should face the floor.

Bunt the ball gently with the tube, trying to keep the ball moving in a straight line.

When you can do this easily, bunt once to the left, then straight in front of you, then to the right, then straight in front of you, etc.

When you can do that easily, turn your body around one complete turn between each bunt so that you end up facing the ball again.

Goal: The ability to control the movement of the ball through space.

14. Dodge Ball

Purpose: To develop good eye-body coordination.

Material: Sponge ball suspended from the ceiling about chest height

Procedure: Stand directly in front of the ball. Have someone hold the ball out as far from you as he can, and then release the ball. The ball will swing toward your chest. Try to move out of the ball's way without moving your feet from the position.

Continuing to look forward, move your torso so that the ball does not hit you on the back swing. When the ball is behind your back, try to visualize its position and speed.

If you do not have anyone to help you, just push the ball away from you to do the exercise.

Goals: Good eye-body coordination.

Good visualization of space and time.

15. Binocular String

Purpose: To become aware of how your two eyes work.

Materials: A piece of string, four feet long

Procedure: Tie one end of the string to your wall at eye level. (The knob on a cabinet is often useful for this.) Hold the string taut so that it reaches the tip of your nose.

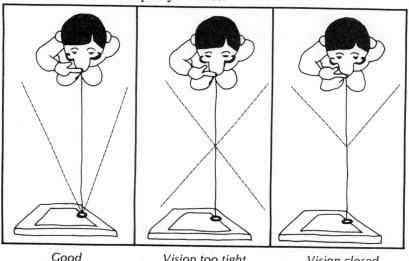

| Good | Vision too tight | Vision closed |

Look carefully at the end of the string near the wall. The string should appear as two strings converging in a "v" toward the wall, if your eyes are aimed correctly at the end of the string. The strings will meet at that place where your eyes are really looking. If your eyes are really looking at a point in space closer than the end of the string, you will not see a "v" but an "x" or a "y" instead. If this is the case, try to relax your looking. Try to look at the end of the string as if you were looking at a point in space farther away. When you are able to look in a relaxed manner, you will be able to look at the end of the string and continue to see a "v" even after opening and closing your eyes several times.

If the strings do not quite come together at the end, concentrate more. Be more critical in looking. Try to see the fuzz on the end of the string more clearly.

When you are successful with this exercise, you should be able to see a "v" anytime you want to.

Goals: To be aware of your two eyes working.

To see how critical or uncritical you are in aiming your eyes.

16. Convergence Training

Purpose: To be able to converge your eyes so that you will be able to concentrate on close visual tasks with comfort.

Materials: Pencil, 3 by 5 card

Procedure: Place a 3 by 5 card on the wall slightly below your eye level.

Stand about 10 feet from the card, with your nose lined up with the card.

Hold a pencil vertically about 16 inches in front of your eyes. The pencil should also be lined up with your nose.

Look at the card. It should appear as one card, but at the same time notice, with the periphery of your vision, that the pencil appears as double images. If you are holding the pencil in line with your nose, each image of the pencil should be an equal distance on either side of the middle of the card. If not, the pencil is not lined up with your nose. Recenter it.

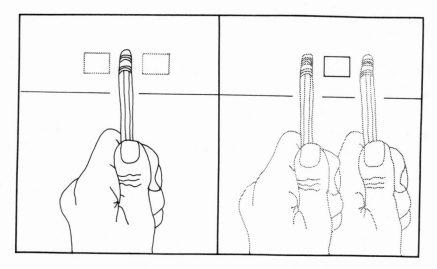

Now shift your gaze to the pencil. It should appear as one pencil. However, the card should appear as double in the periphery of your vision. They should be framing the pencil, equally on each side.

Shift your vision from pencil to card, back to pencil, etc.

Each time the object you are concentrating on should appear single with the other as double.

After doing this successfully a few times, move the pencil one inch closer and repeat. Continue this until the pencil is approximately three inches from your nose.

Note, also as you do this exercise, what happens to the separation of the double image. What does this tell you about accurately perceiving objects in space? The greater the separation, the farther the object is from the area you are concentrating on.

Be careful that your posture is relaxed and appropriate. Any tilting of your head will show up as one double image being higher than the other.

Goal: Be able to easily shift back and forth from a distant target to a near one without distorting your posture.

17. Simple Fusion

Purpose: To develop simple fusion (the blending of colors).

Materials: Mirror, two 8 by 10 sheets of construction paper, one red and one green.

Procedure: Stand in a corner of your room so that one wall is 20 inches in front of your eyes and the side wall is 20 inches from your ear.

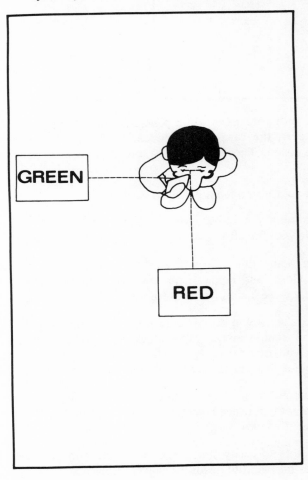

Place the red paper on the wall in front of your eyes about eye level.

Place the green paper on the side wall opposite your ear.

Take a small mirror and place it against your nose so that you can look into the mirror with the eye nearest the side wall and see the green paper reflected in the mirror.

The other eye should be free to look straight ahead and see the red paper.

If you gently angle the mirror, you should see the red paper appearing to blend with the green paper.

Try to see an equal mixture of colors for as long as you can.

Repeat the exercise in a different corner of your room so that you can use the mirror angled in front of your other eye.

Goal: Easy color fusion (blending of two colors).

18. Pumpkin Fusion

Purpose: To help develop the ability to concentrate visually.

Materials: Two identical drawings of a pumpkin face, pointer (tip of a sharp pencil can be used)

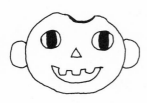
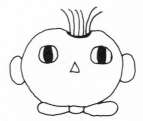

Procedure: Place the two pumpkin faces on a table, at the same level, about 2 inches apart from each other. The pumpkins should be facing the same direction.

Sit comfortably in front of the pumpkins.

Hold the pointer so that the tip rests on the table between the pumpkins.

Concentrate on the tip of the pointer. Out of the corner of your vision be aware of the pumpkins.

Slowly move the pointer toward your nose. *Continue to concentrate on the tip of the pointer.*

When the pointer gets about eight inches off the table, you should notice through your peripheral vision that first the pumpkins appear to double (to four pumpkins) and then the two center pumpkins merge into *one complete pumpkin.*

You now see three pumpkins. The original left one, the merged center ones, and the original right one.

Concentrate on the place in *space* where the tip of the pointer is as you remove the actual pointer from your view.

When you can do this successfully, you will still see three pumpkins.

Look off into space to relax your eyes and then back to that close point in space—imagine where the pointer was—and regain the three pumpkins.

If you cannot do this without the pointer, start the procedure again with the aid of the pointer.

Goal: The ability to concentrate visually on a place in space without any physical aid.

19. Three Coin Magic

Purpose: To help develop the ability to concentrate visually.

Materials: Two identical coins, pointer (tip of sharp pencil can be used)

Procedure: Place the two coins on a table, at the same level, about 2 inches apart from each other. The coins should have the same pictures and face the same direction.

Sit comfortably in front of the coins.

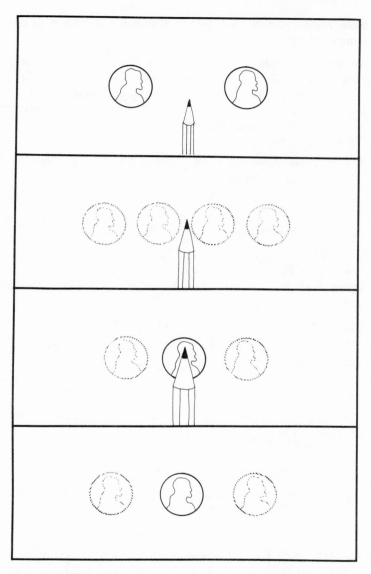

Hold the pointer so that the tip rests on the table between the coins.

Concentrate on the tip of the pointer. Out of the corner of your vision, be aware of the coins.

Slowly move the pointer toward your nose. *Continue to concentrate on the tip of the pointer.*

As you bring the pointer off the table by about 8 inches, you should notice through your peripheral vision that, at first, the coins appeared to double (to four coins), and then the center coins finally merge into one. At that point you should have been aware of the merged coin and the two other coins, one on either side of the merged coin.

You now see three coins: the original left one, the merged one, and the original right one.

Concentrate on the place in *space* where the tip of the pointer is, as you remove the actual pointer from your view. When you can do this successfully you will still see three coins.

Look off into space now to relax your eyes, and then back to that close point in space where the pointer *was,* and regain sight of the three coins.

If you cannot do this without the pointer, start the procedure again with the aid of the pointer.

Goal: The ability to concentrate visually on a place in space without any physical aid.

20. Visual Memory

Purpose: To develop a visual memory for shapes.

Materials: 10 cards, approximately 3 by 3 inches. On each, draw designs similar to the following examples:

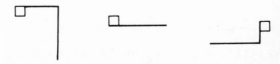

Procedure: Turn the cards face down.

Turn the first card over, and as you say "Look" out loud turn it face down again.

Try to see the picture in your mind's eye without *verbally* describing it to yourself.

Try to hold the mind's eye picture as you draw the shapes on another piece of paper. If you are really good at keeping the picture in your mind's eye, it will look to you as if you are tracing the shapes on the paper.

Turn the card over again and check your accuracy. If you were correct, go on to the next card. If not, look again at the card—without *verbally* describing it to yourself—and then turn it over and correct your drawing.

If you are consistently able to draw seven out of 10 correctly on the first look, make up a new series. If not, shuffle the cards. Since they are square you can rotate each card so that you have 40 choices, 10 cards, 4 positions each.

When you are good at the first series, try these:

Series two:

When good at series two, try:

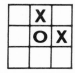 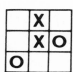 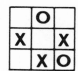

Series three:

21. Visualizing Body Movements

Purpose: To be able to visualize your body's position from a code.

Materials: Body code sheet, metronome or record with a good beat.

Procedure: Place the code sheet in front of you so that it is easily visible.

CODE 1

Set your metronome on 60 beats a minute, or play a record.

Stand in a comfortable position.

Starting at the top left and reading to the right, at each beat imitate the body position shown in the code.

When you are good at code #1, proceed to 2, 3, 4.

When you can do all of them easily, make up your own code by combining all four.

Body Code

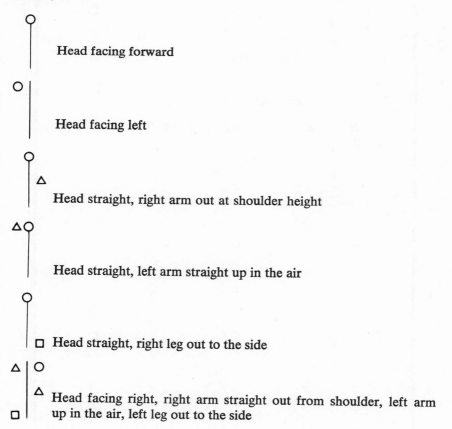

Head facing forward

Head facing left

Head straight, right arm out at shoulder height

Head straight, left arm straight up in the air

Head straight, right leg out to the side

Head facing right, right arm straight out from shoulder, left arm up in the air, left leg out to the side

Goal: To easily follow the body code, at the beat, with a minimum of effort.

CODE 2

CODE 3

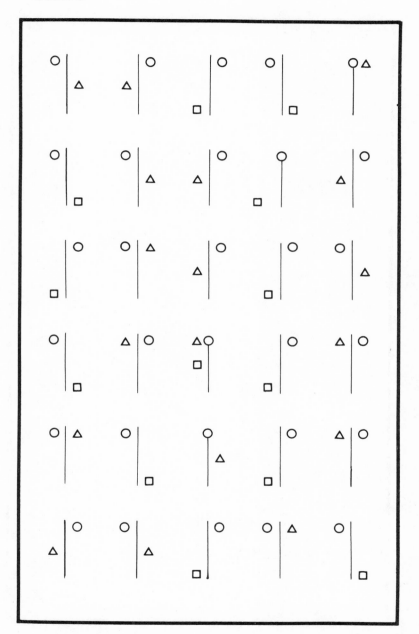

CODE 4

22. Scene Visualization

Purpose: To extend the ability to see with the mind's eye.

Materials: None

Procedure: Picture in your mind's eye a place that you frequently visit, such as a favorite store, etc.

Imagine walking into the store. Imagine with your whole body. What do you do? Do you push the door in? Out? Turn the knob? How does it feel?

Walk in through the door two steps, four steps, 10 steps. Turn to your right, your left, look straight ahead of you. What do you see?

Reach out to your left and right. What does your hand touch? How does it feel?

Go to the store or other place you were thinking of and check your visualizations.

Goal: To imagine being in a familiar place and re-experience it.

23. Roving Artist

Purpose: To visualize what a scene would look like if you viewed it from a different position.

Materials: Paper and pencil, various objects.

Procedure: Set up two or three objects in front of you. Sketch their relative positions.

Now *mentally* walk around the objects to another position. Sketch the objects as you would see them if you actually did move to this position.

After you finish your sketch, walk around the objects to that position and check your sketch.

If you are correct, try another position. If you are incorrect, walk back to the starting position and try to revisualize what you had previously seen.

Sketch and check again.

Goal: To be able to visualize being in another place.

24. Visual Scanning

Purpose: To be able quickly and easily to scan a field of information in an organized manner.

Materials: Scan sheet, timer.

Procedure: Place the scan sheet in front of you. Note when the second hand of your watch is on twelve. Note also where the minute hand is.

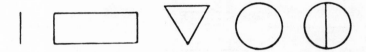

Quickly scan the sheet in an organized manner as you count how many of each object there are.

Mark down the number.

When you are finished, check your answers.

When you can scan the pattern in 20 seconds, then try it with the following changes in the count:

a) each ⊕ counts 2, as does each △ .

b)   −3,   −2,   −4.

Scan Sheet-count one for each figure

Goals: To be able to scan the pattern easily and accurately in 20 seconds, picking out one kind of figure.

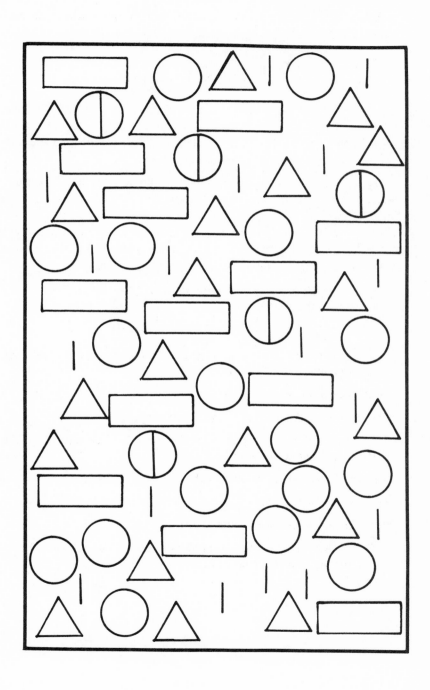

25. Visualizing Time and Distance

Purpose: To be able to see, in your mind's eye, the way to solve a problem.

Materials: Metronome, a string 12 feet long, various objects of different weights.

Procedure: Hang the string from a height and tie an object to the end of it. The object should be able to freely swing back and forth.

Try to visualize how you can arrange the string (length, weight, amount of push, etc.) to match the speed of the metronome.

Use varying metronome speeds.

What is the relationship?

What picture or symbol do you see in your mind's eye?

Try this game with children of different ages and observe how they picture the solution.

26. Expand Your Perceptual Awareness

Purpose: To increase your visual volume (your ability to attend to many things without being distracted).

Materials: Central target to fixate, movable peripheral targets.

Procedure: Place your fixation target in front of you at eye level. Cut out and arrange on the wall in random order the figures on the bottom of this page (or use other shapes of your own design).

As you look steadily at the fixation target, become aware out of the corners of your eyes of the peripheral targets and their relative sizes.

Take a pencil and lightly mark them from 1-10 according to their size (#1 smallest, #10 largest), as you continue to look at the fixation target.

Repeat the marking several times until you feel confident of your ability to estimate their relative sizes.

Goal: To estimate accurately peripheral targets, no matter what their positions.

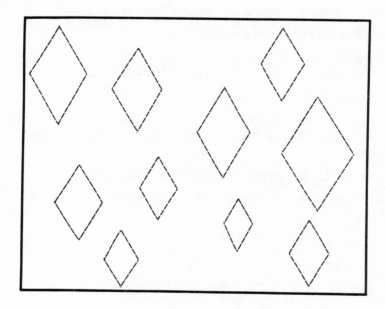

27. Visual Classifications

Purpose: To be able to reclassify objects and events quickly.

Materials: Five blue, red, yellow circles.

Four blue, red, yellow squares.

Six blue, yellow large triangles.

Procedure: Place all pieces in front of you.

As quickly as you can, sort the pieces into groups with common attributes (e.g. all circles).

When you are finished, try to quickly re-sort the pieces into different categories.

Goal: To flexibly change your grouping and classifying.

Note: Nine categories is the average. How many do you see?

28. Sight Improvement

Purpose: To improve your ability to see objects in the distance.

Materials: Letter chart (or a calendar)

Procedure: Look at the top line of letters and slowly back away until they can no longer be seen. Take an additional step.

Tighten both fists very hard.

Lean forward at the waist and blink rapidly. Move forward slowly until you can just barely see the letters, even though they are blurred.

Relax. Breathe deeply several times and start again.

Goal: To see at further distances when you and your body are *relaxed*.

29. Quick Wink

Purpose: To see details clearly by the help of background objects and peripheral vision.

Materials: Letter chart (or calendar).

Procedure: Look *toward* the letters, not *at* them.

Be aware at all times of the surrounding area.

Inhale quickly, block the intake, and blink without moving your eyes from the target.

Relax.

Breathe again normally, while you call out the smallest letters that you can see. Skip any letters which do not immediately emerge from the blur.

Goal: To see objects more clearly.

Appendix:
Finding a Behavioral Optometrist

If you have any difficulty finding a behavioral optometrist, contact the following agencies for advice:

American Optometric Association
Attn: Chairman, Vision Training Committee
7000 Chippiewa Street
St. Louis, Missouri 63119

Local Optometric Society
e.g., New York Optometric Society

American Academy of Optometry
Attn: Chairman of the Diplomate Program in Binocular Vision
    and Perception
118 North Oak Street
Owatonna, Minnesota 55060

Optometric Extension Program
Duncan, Oklahoma 73533

College of Optometrists in Vision Development
353 H Street, Suite C
Chula Vista, California 92010

Optometry colleges:

Illinois College of Optometry
3241 South Michigan Avenue
Chicago, Illinois 60616

Indiana University School of Optometry
Bloomington, Indiana 47401

Ferris State College of Optometry
Big Rapids, Michigan 49307

New England College of Optometry
424 Beacon Street
Boston, Massachusetts 02115

The Ohio State University
College of Optometry
338 West 10th Street
Columbus, Ohio 43210

The Pacific University College of Optometry
Forest Grove, Oregon 97116

Pennsylvania College of Optometry
1200 West Godfrey Avenue
Philadelphia, Pennsylvania 19141

Southern California College of Optometry
2001 Associated Road
Fullerton, California 92631

State University of New York
State College of Optometry
122 East 25th Street
New York, New York 10010

University of California
School of Optometry
Berkeley, California 94720

University of Houston
College of Optometry
Houston, Texas 77004

University of Montreal
School of Optometry
B.O. 6128
Montreal, Quebec H3C 3J7
Canada

University of Waterloo
School of Optometry
Waterloo, Ontario N2L 3G1
Canada

Bibliography

General Information

Arena, John I., ed. "Successful Programming: Many Points of View." In *Proceedings of the Fifth Annual Conference of the Association for Children with Learning Disabilities*. San Rafael, California: Academic Therapy Publications, 1969.

Beadle, Muriel. *A Child's Mind*. New York: Anchor Books, 1971.

Bower, T. G. R. *A Primer of Infant Development*. San Francisco: Freeman, 1977.

Doman, G. *What To Do About Your Brain Injured Child*. Garden City, New York: Doubleday & Company, 1974.

Ebersole, Mary Lou; Kephart, Newell C.; and Ebersole, James B. *Steps to Achievement for the Slow Learner*. Columbus, Ohio: Charles E. Merrill Books, 1971.

Ellingson, Careth. *The Shadow Children: A Book about Children's Learning Disorders*. Chicago: Topaz Books, 1967.

Flowers, Ann M. *Helping the Child with a Learning Disability*. Danville, Illinois: Interstate Printers & Publishers, 1969.

Gesell, Arnold. *The Child from Five to Ten*. New York: Harper & Row, 1949.

————. *The First Five Years of Life*. New York: Harper & Row, 1946.

————. *Youth: Years from Ten to Sixteen*. New York: Harper & Row, 1956.

Gesell et al. *Infant and Child in the Culture of Today*. New York: Harper & Row, 1943.

Getman, G. N. *How to Develop Your Child's Intelligence*. Luverne, Minnesota: The Announcer Press, 1958.

Goldstein, Kurt. *The Organism*. New York: American Book Co., 1939.

Gregg, James R., and Heath, Gordon. *The Eye and Sight*. Boston: D. C. Heath and Co.

Gregory, R. L. *Eye and Brain*. New York: World University Library/ McGraw-Hill, 1966.

————. *The Intelligent Eye*. New York: McGraw-Hill, 1970.

Haeusserman, E. *Developmental Potential of Preschool Children*. New York: Grune & Stratton, 1958.

Hart, Jane, and Jones, Beverly. *Where's Hannah?* New York: Hart Publishing Co., 1968.

Hebb, D. O. *The Organization of Behavior*. New York: John Wiley and Sons, 1939.

Ilg, Francis L., and Ames, L. B. *School Readiness*. New York: Harper & Row, 1964.

————. *Parents Ask*. Laurel Edition. New York: Dell Books, 1965.

————. *The Gesell Institute's Child Behavior*. New York: Dell Books, 1955.

Kitchell, Frank M. *Opportunities in an Optometric Career*. New York: Vocational Guidance Manuals, 1967.

Lambeth, J. *What Optometry and Its Related Fields Have to Offer the Reading Teacher*. Duncan, Oklahoma: Optometric Extension Program Foundation, 1966.

Levy, H. *Square Pegs, Round Holes*. Boston: Little, Brown and Company, 1973.

Liepman, Lisé. *Your Child's Sensory World*. New York: Dial Press, 1973.

Norris, Ralph C., and Gibson, Robert C. *Learning Disabilities: A Handbook for Parents and Teachers*. Des Moines, Iowa: Iowa Association for Children with Learning Disabilities, 1970.

Orem, R. *Developmental Vision for Lifelong Learning*. Johnstown, Pennsylvania: Mafex Association, 1977.

————. *A Montessori Handbook*. New York: G. P. Putnam's Sons, 1965.

————. *Montessori and the Special Child*. New York: G. P. Putnam's Sons, 1969.

Radler, D. H., and Kephart, Newell C. *Success through Play*. New York: Harper & Row, 1960.

Rosner, J. *Helping Children Overcome Learning Difficulties*. New York: Walker & Co., 1975.

Simpson, Dorothy M. *Learning to Learn*. Columbus, Ohio: Charles E. Merrill Books, Inc., 1972.

Sneller, Robert C. *Vision and Driving*. St. Louis, Missouri: American Optometric Association, 1969.

Stuart, Marion. *Neurophysiological Insights into Teaching*. Palo Alto, California: Pacific Books, 1963.

Wunderlich, Ray C. *Kids, Brains and Learning*. St. Petersburg, Florida: Johnny Reads, 1970.

Philosophy

Books

Apell, R. J. and Lowry, R. W. *Preschool Vision*. St. Louis: American Optometric Association, 1959.

Bartley, S. Howard. *The Human Organism as a Person*. Philadelphia: Chilton, 1967.

Delacato, Carl H. *Neurological Organization and Reading*. Springfield, Illinois: Charles C. Thomas, 1966.

————. *The Diagnosis and Treatment of Speech and Reading Problems*. Springfield, Illinois: Charles C. Thomas, 1965.

Frostig, Marianne, and Horne, David. *The Frostig Program for the Development of Visual Perception*. Chicago: Follett Publishing Co., 1964.

Gesell, Arnold. *The Embryology of Behavior*. New York: Harper & Row, 1945.

————. *Infant Development*. New York: Harper & Row, 1952.

Gesell, Arnold; Ilg, Francis L.; and Bullis, G. E. *Vision: Its Development in Infant and Child*. 1949. Reprint. New York: Hafner, 1967.

Getman, G. N. *Techniques and Diagnostic Criteria for the Optometric Care of Children's Vision*. Duncan, Oklahoma: Optometric Extension Program Foundation, Inc., 1960.

Getman, G. N.; Kane, Elmer R.; Halgren, Marvin A.; and McKee, Gordon W. *Developing Learning Readiness: A Visual-Motor-Tactile Skills Program*. St. Louis: Webster Division of McGraw-Hill, Inc., 1968.

Harmon, D. B. *Dynamic Theory of Vision*. Austin, Texas: Research Press, 1959.

Hirsch, Monroe J., and Wick, Ralph E., eds. *Vision of Children: An Optometric Symposium*. Philadelphia: Chilton, 1963.

Ilg, Francis L., and Ames, Louise B. *School Readiness: Behavior Test Used at the Gesell Institute, New Haven, Conn*. New York: Harper & Row, 1965.

Kephart, Newell C. *The Slow Learner in the Classroom*. Columbus, Ohio: Merrill Books, 1960.

Kraskin, Robert A. *You Can Improve Your Vision.* Garden City, New York: Doubleday & Co., Inc., 1968.

Lambath, Joanne. *What Optometry and Its Related Fields Have To Offer the Reading Teacher.* Duncan, Oklahoma: Optometric Extension Program, 1966.

Orem, E. C., ed. *Learning to See and Seeing to Learn: A Brighter Way of Life for All Children.* Johnstown, Pennsylvania: Mafex Associates, 1971.

Schaffel, Adrienne. *Vision Training: A New Developmental Concept in Child Vision.* Duncan, Oklahoma: Optometric Extension Program, 1972.

Smith, K. U., and Smith, W. M. *Perception and Motion.* Philadelphia: W. B. Saunders Company, 1962.

Wold, Robert M. *Visual Perceptual Aspects for the Achieving and Underachieving Child.* Seattle: Special Child Publications, 1969.

Articles

Baldwin, William R. "Optometry: Child Development and Educability." *Journal of the American Optometry Association* 40 (February 1969): 131–133.

Cohen, S. A. "A Dynamic Theory of Vision." *The Journal of Developmental Reading* 6 (Autumn 1962): 15–25.

Flax, Nathan. "Problems in Relating Visual Function to Reading Disorder." *American Journal of Optometry and Archives of American Academy of Optometry* 47 (May 1970): 366–372.

————. "Visual Function in Dyslexia." *American Journal of Optometry and Archives of American Academy of Optometry* 45 (September 1968): 574–587.

Getman, G. N. and Streff, John W. "Mommy and Daddy, You Can Help Me Learn to See." Duncan, Oklahoma: Optometric Extension Program, Women's Auxiliary to the American Optometric Association, 1959.

Harmon, Darell Boyd. "Controlling the Thermal Environment of the Coordinated Classroom." Monograph. Minneapolis, Minn. Minneapolis Honeywell Regulator Company, 1954.

————. "Coordinated Classroom." *The Nation's Schools* (March 1950).

Heinsen, Arthur C. "Concept and Scope of Developmental Optometry." *Journal of the American Optometric Association* 40 (November 1969): 1088–1093.

Hendrikson, Homer H. "The Vision Development Process." Duncan, Oklahoma: Optometric Extension Program Foundation, 1969.

Hoffman, Leon; Cohen, Allen H.; and Feuer, Gary. "Effectiveness of Non-Strabismus Optometric Vision Training in a Private Practice." *American Journal of Optometry and Archives of the American Academy of Optometry* 50 (October 1973): 813–816.

Kirshner, A. J. "Developmental Optometry and Physiological Optics." *Journal of the American Optometric Association* 38 (October 1967): 851–852.

Manas, Leo. "The Optometric Approach to Gross Motor Training." *Association for Physical and Mental Rehabilitation, now American Corrective Therapy Association Journal.* Chicago Circle Campus, March 22–23, 1967.

McKee, Gordon W. "The Role of the Optometrist in the Development of Perceptual and Visuomotor Skills in Children." *American Journal of Optometry and Archives of the American Academy of Optometry* 44 (May 1967): 297–310.

Mullins, June B. "A Rationale for Visual Training: The Role of the Optometrist from the Standpoint of Special Education and Rehabilitation." *Journal of the American Optometric Association* 40 (February 1969): 139–143.

Swanson, William L. "Optometric Vision Therapy: How Successful Is It in the Treatment of Learning Disorders?" *Journal of Learning Disabilities* 5 (May 1972): 285–290.

Physiology

Alexander, F. Matthias. *Resurrection of the Body.* New York: University Books, Inc., 1969.

Anderson, T. M. *Human Kinetics and Analyses of Body Movements.* London: William Heinemann Medical Books, 1951.

Birdwhistell, Ray L. *Kinesics and Context.* New York: Ballantine Books, 1972.

Cannon, W. B. *The Wisdom of the Body.* New York: W. W. Norton, 1932.

Chalfant, James C., and Scheffelin, Margaret A. *Central Processing Dysfunctions in Children: A Review of Research.* Bethesda, Maryland: U.S. Department of Health, Education and Welfare, 1969.

Duke, Elder. *System of Ophthalmology.* Vol. 6. Ocular Motility and Strabismus. St. Louis: C. V. Mosby Company, 1973.

Dunbar, Helen Flanders. *Emotions and Bodily Changes.* New York: Columbia University Press, 1935.

Fisher, Seymour. *Body Consciousness—You Are What You Feel.* Englewood Cliffs, New Jersey: Prentice-Hall, Inc., 1973.

Gaarder, K. *Eye Movements, Vision and Behavior.* New York: John Wiley & Sons, Inc., 1975.

Gay, A. J.; Newman, M. M.; Keltner, J. L.; and Stroud, M. H. *Eye Movement Disorders.* St. Louis: C. V. Mosby Company, 1974.

Gunther, Bernard. *Sense Relaxation.* New York: The Macmillan Company, 1968.

Helmuth, J., ed. *Exceptional Infant—The Normal Infant.* New York: Brunner-Mazel, 1967.

Jacobson, Edmund. *Progressive Relaxation.* Chicago: University of Chicago Press, 1938.

Kestenberg, Judith. *The Role of Movement Patterns in Development.* New York: Dance Notation Bureau, 1967.

Lowen, Alexander. *The Betrayal of the Body.* London: Collier Macmillan, 1967.

———. *Depression and the Body.* Baltimore, Maryland: Penguin Books, 1972.

Ludlam, William M. "Review of the Psychophysiological Factors in Visual Information Processing as They Relate to Learning." In *Vision and Learning Disabilities,* edited by Tole N. Greenstein, pp. 179–222. St. Louis: American Optometric Association, 1976.

North, Marion. *Movement Education: Child Development Through Body Motion.* New York: E. P. Dutton & Co., 1973.

———. *Body Movement for Children.* Boston: Plays, 1971.

Riesen, A. *The Developmental Neuropsychology of Sensory Deprivation.* New York: Academic Press, 1975.

Selye, Hans. *The Story of the Adaptation Syndrome.* Montreal: Acta, Inc., Medical Publishers, 1952.

———. *The Stress of Life.* New York: McGraw-Hill, 1956.

Psychology

Books

Bannatype, Alex, and Maryl. *The Body Image/Communication Psycho-Physical Development Program.* Miami: Kismet Publishing Co., 1976.

Chess, Stella. *An Introduction to Child Psychiatry.* New York: Grune and Stratton, 1969.

Cleveland, S. E., and Fisher, S. *Body Image and Personality*. Princeton, New Jersey: D. Van Nostrand Company, Inc., 1958.

Corballis, M., and Beale, I. *The Psychology of Left and Right*. New York: John Wiley & Sons, 1976.

Eliot, S., and Salkind, N. *Children's Spatial Development*. Springfield, Illinois: Chas. Thomas, 1975.

Flavell, J. *The Developmental Psychology of Jean Piaget*. Princeton, New Jersey: D. Van Nostrand Company, Inc., 1964.

Gesell, A., and Amatruda, C. *Developmental Diagnosis*. New York: Hoeber Division, Harper & Row, 1941.

Gesell, A.; Thompson, H.; and Armatruda, C. *The Psychopathology of Early Growth Including Norms of Infant Behavior and a Method of Genetic Analysis*. New York: Macmillan, 1938.

Harris, Dale B. *Children's Drawings as Measures of Intellectual Maturity: A Revision and Extension of the Goodenough Draw-A-Man Test*. New York: Harcourt, Brace & World, 1963.

Kogan, N. *Cognitive Style in Early Infancy and Early Childhood*. New York: John Wiley & Sons, 1976.

Koppitz, Elizabeth Munsterberg. *The Bender-Gestalt Test for Young Children*. New York: Grune and Stratton, 1964.

Laurendean, Monique, and Pinard, Adrien. *The Development of the Concept of Space in the Child*. New York: International Universities Press, 1970.

Lipsitt, Lewis P. *Advances in Child Development and Behavior*. Vols. 1 and 2. Edited by Charles C. Spiker. New York: Academic Press, 1963.

Martin, William E., and Stendler, Celia Burns. *Child Behavior and Development*. New York: Harcourt, Brace & World, 1959.

Perls, Frederick. *Ego, Hunger and Aggression*. New York: Random House, Inc., 1969.

———. *Gestalt Therapy Verbatim*. Lafayette, California: Real People Press, 1969.

Perls, Frederick; Hefferline, Ralph F.; and Goodman, Paul. *Gestalt Therapy*. New York: Delta Books, 1965.

Renshaw, S. *Psychological Optics*. Vols. 10, 11, 12. Duncan, Oklahoma: Optometric Extension Program, 1950–1951.

Schilder, Paul. *The Image and Appearance of the Human Body*. New York: International University Press, 1950.

———. *Brain and Personality*. Monograph Series No. 53. New York: Nervous and Mental Diseases Publishing Company, 1931.

Articles

Ball, Thomas S., and Edgar, Olav Lee. "The Effectiveness of Sensory-Motor Training in Promoting Generalized Body Image Development." *Journal of Special Education* 1 (Summer 1967): 387–395.

Koppitz, Elizabeth Munsterberg. "Brain Damage, Reading Disability and the Bender-Gestalt Test." *Journal of Learning Disabilities* 3 (September 1970): 429–433.

Mittler, P. "The Use of Form Boards in Developmental Assessment." *Developmental Medicine and Child Neurology* 6: (1964).

Swanson, Robert, and Benton, Arthur L. "Some Aspects of the Genetic Development of Right-Left Discrimination." *Child Development* 26 (1955): 123–133.

Therapy

Books

Giles, G. *The Practice of Orthoptics*. London: Hammond, Hammond & Co., 1945.

Griffin, J. *Binocular Anomalies: Procedures for Vision Therapy*. Chicago: Professional Press, 1976.

Kavner, R., and Suchoff, I. *Pleoptics Handbook*. New York: New York State University Press, 1972.

Articles

Amble, Bruce R. "Phrase Reading Development: The Enhancement of Reading Skills through Perceptual Span Training." In *Visual and Perceptual Aspects for the Achieving and Underachieving Child,* edited by Robert M. Wold, pp. 281–293. Seattle: Special Child Publications, 1969.

Beach, G., and Kavner, R. "Conjoint Therapy: A Co-operative Psycho-therapeutic-Optometric Approach to Therapy." *Journal of the American Optometric Association,* December 1977, pp. 1501–1507.

Cooper, Jeffrey S., and Baron, Samuel J. "Treatment of a Divergence Excess and Amblyopia with Orthoptic Training and Contact Lenses." *Journal of the American Optometric Association* 45 (June 1974): 743–745.

Cox, Brian J., and Hambly, Lionel R. "Guided Development of Perceptual Skill of Visual Space as a Factor in the Achievement of

Primary Grade Children." *American Journal of Optometry and Archives of the American Academy of Optometry* 38 (August 1961): 433–444.

Crow, George, and Fuog, H. L. "Fundamental Principles of Visual Training." Series 8. Duncan, Oklahoma: Optometric Extension Program, 1958–1959.

Getman, G. N., and Kephart, N. C. "Developmental Vision." Series 2, nos. 10, 12, 1957–1958; Series 3, nos. 1–12, 1958–1959. Duncan, Oklahoma: Optometric Extension Program.

Griffin, John R. "Pursuit Fixations: An Overview of Training Procedures." *The Optometric Weekly* 67 (13 May 1976): 534–537.

Hoffman, Leon, and Cohen, Allen H. "A Developmental View of Visual Therapy." *Journal of the American Optometric Association* 39 (January 1968): 44–47.

Kavner, R. "Minimal Brain Damage—An Overview and Rationale for Optometric Care." *Optical Journal and Review of Optometry,* 15 September 1968, pp. 33–41.

Kavner, R., and Suchoff, I. "Occlusion Techniques in Amblyopia." *Optical Journal and Review of Optometry,* 1 April 1964, pp. 25–27.

———. "Pleoptic Evaluation." *Optical Journal and Review of Optometry,* 1 March 1964, pp. 21–24.

———. "Pleoptics—Background and Philosophy." *Optical Journal and Review of Optometry,* 15 February 1964, pp. 29–32.

———. "Pleoptics: Case Studies—Supplementary Notes." *Optical Journal and Review of Optometry,* 15 August 1964, pp. 27–31.

———. "Pleoptic Techniques, Part I." *Optical Journal and Review of Optometry,* 1 June 1964, pp. 23–27.

———. "Pleoptic Techniques, Part II." *Optical Journal and Review of Optometry,* 15 June 1964, pp. 31–34.

Kraskin, Robert A. "Variations on Basic Techniques." Vol. 5, no. 6. Optometric Extension Program. Duncan, Oklahoma, 1956.

Lowry, Raymond W., Jr. "Equipment-Books about the Reading Method." 1963. Series 1, no. 3, p. 17. Optometric Extension Program. Duncan, Oklahoma.

Ludlam, William M.; Twaraski, Chester; and Ludlam, Diana T. "Optometric Visual Training for Reading Disability: A Case Report." *American Journal of Optometry and Archives of the American Academy of Optometry* 59 (January 1973): 58–66.

Lyons, C. V.; and Lyons, E. B. "The Power of Visual Training as Measured in Factors of Intelligence." *The Journal of the American Optometric Association,* December 1954, pp. 255–262.

————. "The Power of Visual Training, Part II. Further Studies Measured in Factors of Intelligence." *Journal of the American Optometric Association* 45 (November 1956): 217–226.

————. "The Power of Optometric Visual Training, Part III: A Loom for Productive Thinking." *Journal of the American Optometric Association* 38 (June 1957): 640–653.

————. "The Power of Visual Training, Part V: A Philosophy of Visualization." *Journal of the American Optometric Association* 38 (August 1967): 654–660.

————. "The Power of Visual Training, Part IV: To Build Minds." *Journal of the American Optometric Association* 32 (June 1961): 879–885.

MacDonald, Lawrence W. "Visual Training." Series 1–3. Optometric Extension Program. Duncan, Oklahoma, 1962–1966.

McCoy, Dorothea M. "Mirror Training Techniques." *Visual Training at Work.* Vol. 4, no. 1, pp. 1–4. Optometric Extension Program. Duncan, Oklahoma, 1954.

Paul, Howard A., and Markow, Michael J. "Neurological Organization Exercises on Retarded Children with Strabismus." *Journal of the American Optometric Association* 40 (July 1969): 706–709.

Renshaw, Samuel. "Tachistoscopic Studies on Visual Perception." Vol. 1, no. 8, p. 1. Optometric Extension Program. Duncan, Oklahoma, 1940.

Spencer, Richard W. "Optometric Handling of Perceptual-Motor Problems." In *Interdisciplinary Approaches to Learning Disorders,* edited by Darrell B. Carter, pp. 141–147. Philadelphia: Chilton Book Company, 1970.

Swanson, William L. "The Role of the Optometrist in the Treatment of Strephosymbolia." In *Visual and Perceptual Aspects for the Achieving and Underachieving Child,* edited by Robert M. Wold, pp. 373–391. Seattle: Special Child Publications, 1969.

Woolf, Daniel. "Visual Function in Theory and Practice." Series 1–4. Optometric Extension Program. Duncan, Oklahoma, 1963–1966.

Strabismus

Articles

Allen, Merrill J. "Strabismus Clinic Progress Report." *Journal of the American Optometric Association* 42 (April 1971): 367–68.

Bietti, G. "Problems of Anesthesia in Strabismus Surgery." *International Ocular Clinics* 6 (1966).

Bonsor, A. "Some Comments on the Question of Early Operation." *British Ophthalmology Journal* 16 (1959): 114–118.

Bridgeman, A. "Convergent Squint of Early Onset—Results of Treatment." *British Ophthalmology Journal* 20 (1963): 45–53.

Costenbader, F. and Albert D. "Surgery of Strabismus." *International Ocular Clinics* 2 (1962).

Dunlap, E. "Complications in Strabismus Surgery." *International Ocular Clinics* 6 (1966).

Fletcher, M., and Silverman, S. "Strabismus, A Study of 1,110 Consecutive Cases." *American Journal of Ophthalmology,* 61, no. 25, pp. 86–94.

Gartner, S., and Billet, E. "A Study of Mortality Rates during General Anesthesia for Ophthalmic Surgery." *American Journal of Ophthalmology,* 45, no. 2, pp. 847–849.

Hardesty, H. "Treatment of Recurrent Intermittent Exotropia." *American Journal of Ophthalmology,* 60, no. 6, pp. 1036–1046.

Hoffman, Leon; Cohen, Allen H.; Fever, Gary; and Klayman, Ivan. "Effectiveness of Optometric Therapy for Strabismus in a Private Practice." *American Journal of Optometry and Archives of the American Academy of Optometry* 47 (December 1970): 990–995.

Kennedy, R., and McCarthy, M. "Surgical Treatment of Esotropia." *American Journal of Ophthalmology* 50 (April 1969): 508–518.

Ludlam, William M. "Orthoptic Treatment of Strabismus." *American Journal of Optometry and Archives of the American Academy of Optometry* 38 (July 1961): 369–388.

Ludlam, William M., and Kleinman, Burton I. "The Long Range Results of Orthoptic Treatment of Strabismus." *American Journal of Optometry and Archives of the American Academy of Optometry* 42 (November 1965): 647–684.

Nauheim, J. "Marginal Keratitis and Corneal Ulceration After Surgery on the Extra Ocular Muscles." *Archives of Ophthalmology* 67 (June 1962): 708–711.

Nutt, A. "Surgery in the Treatment of Concomitant Strabismus." *Transactions of the Ophthalmology Society of the United Kingdom* 81 (1961).

Reed, H., and McCaughey, T. "Cardiac Slowing during Strabismus Surgery." *British Journal of Ophthalmology* 46 (1962).

Rhode, J., et al. "A Study of the Electrocardiographic Alterations Occurring during Operations on the Extraocular Muscles." *American Journal of Ophthalmology* 46 (1958): 367–382.

Ruedeman, A. "Foveal Coordination." *American Journal of Ophthalmology* 36 (1953): 1220–1224.

Sorenson, L., and Gilmore, J. "Cardiac Arrest during Strabismus Surgery." *American Journal of Ophthalmology* 41 (1956): 748–752.

Wick, Bruce. "Visual Therapy for Small Angle Esotropia." *American Journal of Optometry and Physiological Optics* 51 (July 1974): 490–496.

Perception

Barsch, R. *Enriching Perception and Cognition*. Vol. 2. Seattle: Special Child Publications, 1968.

Bartley, Howard S. *Principles of Perception*. New York: Harper & Row.

Cohen, A., Salapatek, F. *Infant Perception from Sensation to Cognition*. Vols. 1 and 2. New York: Academic Press, 1975.

Cratty, Bryant J. *Perceptual-Motor Behavior and Educational Processes*. Springfield, Illinois: Charles C. Thomas, 1969.

Gibson, Eleanor J. *Principles of Perceptual Learning and Development*. New York: Appleton-Century-Crofts, 1969.

Gibson, James S. *The Perception of the Visual World*. Boston: Houghton Mifflin Co., 1950.

Hirst, R. J. *Perception and the External World*. New York: The Macmillan Co.

Kidd, Aline H., and Rivoire, Jeanne L., eds. *Perceptual Development in Children*. New York: International Universities Press, 1966.

LeGrand, Yves. *Forms and Space Vision*. Bloomington, Indiana: Indiana University Press, 1967.

Piaget, Jean. *The Mechanisms of Perception*. New York: Basic Books, 1969.

Wohlwill, Joachim F., and Wiener, Morton. "Discrimination of Form Orientation in Young Children." *Child Development* 35 (1964): 1113–1125.

Yarbus, Alfred L. "Eye Movements during Perception of Complex Objects." In *Eye Movements and Vision,* pp. 171–197. New York: Plenum Press, 1967.

Zaporazhets, A. V. "The Development of Perception in the Preschool

Child." In *European Research in Cognitive Development*, edited by T. H. Mussen, pp. 82–101. Monographs of the Society for Research in Child Development, 30, Series no. 100 (1963).

Color

Birren, Faber. *Color Psychology and Color Therapy*. Secaucus, New Jersey: University Books, 1950.

Clark, Linda. *Color Therapy*. Old Greenwich, Connecticut: Devin-Adair, 1975.

Don, Frank. *Color Your World*. New York: Warner/Destiny, 1977.

Luscher, Max, and Scott, Ian. *The Luscher Color Test*. New York: Random House, 1969.

Worthy, Morgan. *Eye Color, Sex and Race*. Anderson, South Carolina: Droke House/Hallus, 1974.

Lighting

Books

Moon, Barry. *Wakefield Lighting—as Flexible as Your Classroom*. New York: Illuminating Engineering, 1949.

Ott, John. *Health & Light*. Old Greenwich, Connecticut: Devon Adair, 1973.

———. *My Ivory Cellar*. Chicago: Twentieth Century Press, 1958.

Seagers, Paul W. *Light, Vision, and Learning*. New York: Better Light Better Sight Bureau, 1963.

Articles

Ott, John. "A Rational Analysis of Ultraviolet as a Vital Part of the Light Spectrum Influencing Photobiological Responses." *Optometric Weekly*, 5 September 1978, pp. 21–30.

———. "The Eyes' Dual Function." *Eye, Ear, Nose and Throat Monthly*. July 1974, pp. 276–281; August 1974, pp. 309–316; September 1974, pp. 377–381.

Peters, R.; Chapin, L.; Leining, K.; and Tucker, H. "Supplemental Lighting Stimulates Growth and Lactation in Cattle." *Science* 199 (February 1978): 911–912.

Nutrition

Borsook, Henry. *Vitamins, What They Are and How They Can Benefit You*. New York: The Viking Press, 1940.

Clark, Linda. *Get Well Naturally*. New York: Arco Press, 1974.

Davis, Adelle. *Let's Eat Right to Keep Fit*. New York: Harcourt Brace Jovanovich, 1965.

Kirschmann, John D. *Nutrition Almanac*. New York: McGraw-Hill, 1975.

Rodale, J. *The Encyclopedia of Common Diseases*. Emmaus, Pennsylvania: Rodale Press, 1976.

————. *The Complete Book of Vitamins*. Emmaus, Pennsylvania: Rodale Press, 1977.

————. *The Natural Way to Better Eyesight*. New York: Pyramid, 1968.

Rosenberg, Harold, and Fedlzamen, A. N. *The Doctor's Book of Vitamin Therapy*. New York: G. P. Putnam's Sons, 1974.

Smith, L. *Improving Your Child's Behavior Chemistry*. Englewood Cliffs, New Jersey: Prentice-Hall, 1976.

Wunderlich, Ray C. *Kids, Brains and Learning*. St. Petersburg, Florida: Johnny Reads Inc., 1970.

Vision and Creativity

Arnheim, Rudolf. *Art and Visual Perception*. Los Angeles: University of California Press, 1954.

————. *Visual Thinking*. London: Faber and Faber, 1969.

Berger, John. *Ways of Seeing*. London: British Broadcasting System and Pelican Books, 1977.

Bloomer, C. *Principles of Visual Perception*. New York: D. Van Nostrand Reinhold Company, 1976.

Dileo, Joseph H. *Young Children and their Drawings*. New York: Brunner/Mazel, 1970.

Hall, Edward T. *The Hidden Dimension*. Garden City, New York: Anchor Books/Doubleday & Company, Inc., 1969.

Kepes, G. *Language of Vision*. Chicago: Paul Theobald Co., 1967.

Lowry, Bates. *The Visual Experience*. Englewood Cliffs, New Jersey: Prentice-Hall, Inc./Harry W. Abrams, 1977.

Trevor-Roper, Patrick. *The World through Blunted Sight.* Indianapolis, Indiana: The Bobbs-Merrill Co., 1970.

Visualizations

Green, Elmer and Alyce. *Beyond Biofeedback.* New York: Delacorte, 1977.

Jung, C. G. *Modern Man in Search of a Soul.* New York: Harcourt, Brace & World, Inc., 1933.

Lawrence, Jodi. *Alpha Brain Waves.* New York: Avon, 1972.

Ostrander, Shelia, and Schroeder, Lynn. *Psychic Discoveries Behind the Iron Curtain.* Englewood Cliffs, New Jersey: Prentice-Hall, Inc., 1970.

Samuels, Mike, and Samuels, Nancy. *Seeing With The Mind's Eye.* New York: Random House; and Berkeley, California: The Bookworks, 1975.

Shorr, Joseph E. *Go See The Movie in Your Head.* New York: Popular Library, 1977.

Smith, Adam. *Powers of Mind.* New York: Random House, 1975.

Index